COPING SUCCESSFULLY WITH PROSTATE CANCER

DR TOM SMITH has been writing full time since 1977, after spending six years in general practice and seven years in medical research. He writes regularly for medical journals and magazines and has a weekly column in the *Bradford Telegraph and Argus*. He also broadcasts regularly for BBC Radio Scotland. His other books for Sheldon Press include *Heart Attacks: Prevent and Survive*, *Living with High Blood Pressure* and *Living with Alzheimer's Disease*.

Overcoming Common Problems Series

For a full list of titles please contact
Sheldon Press, Marylebone Road, London NW1 4DU

Antioxidants
Dr Robert Youngson

The Assertiveness Workbook
Joanna Gutmann

Beating the Comfort Trap
Dr Windy Dryden and Jack Gordon

Body Language
Allan Pease

Body Language in Relationships
David Cohen

Calm Down
Dr Paul Hauck

Cancer – A Family Affair
Neville Shone

The Cancer Guide for Men
Helen Beare and Neil Priddy

The Candida Diet Book
Karen Brody

Caring for Your Elderly Parent
Julia Burton-Jones

Cider Vinegar
Margaret Hills

Comfort for Depression
Janet Horwood

Considering Adoption?
Sarah Biggs

Coping Successfully with Hay Fever
Dr Robert Youngson

Coping Successfully with Pain
Neville Shone

Coping Successfully with Panic Attacks
Shirley Trickett

Coping Successfully with PMS
Karen Evennett

Coping Successfully with Prostate Problems
Rosy Reynolds

Coping Successfully with RSI
Maggie Black and Penny Gray

Coping Successfully with Your Hiatus Hernia
Dr Tom Smith

Coping Successfully with Your Irritable Bladder
Dr Jennifer Hunt

Coping Successfully with Your Irritable Bowel
Rosemary Nicol

Coping When Your Child Has Special Needs
Suzanne Askham

Coping with Anxiety and Depression
Shirley Trickett

Coping with Blushing
Dr Robert Edelmann

Coping with Bronchitis and Emphysema
Dr Tom Smith

Coping with Candida
Shirley Trickett

Coping with Chronic Fatigue
Trudie Chalder

Coping with Coeliac Disease
Karen Brody

Coping with Cystitis
Caroline Clayton

Coping with Depression and Elation
Dr Patrick McKeon

Coping with Eczema
Dr Robert Youngson

Coping with Endometriosis
Jo Mears

Coping with Epilepsy
Fiona Marshall and
Dr Pamela Crawford

Coping with Fibroids
Mary-Claire Mason

Coping with Gallstones
Dr Joan Gomez

Coping with Headaches and Migraine
Shirley Trickett

Coping with a Hernia
Dr David Delvin

Coping with Long-Term Illness
Barbara Baker

Coping with the Menopause
Janet Horwood

Coping with Psoriasis
Professor Ronald Marks

Coping with Rheumatism and Arthritis
Dr Robert Youngson

Overcoming Common Problems Series

Overcoming Common Problems Series

Overcoming Common Problems

Coping Successfully with Prostate Cancer

Dr Tom Smith

sheldon PRESS

Published in Great Britain in 2002 by
Sheldon Press
Holy Trinity Church
Marylebone Road
London NW1 4DU

© Dr Tom Smith 2002

British Library Cataloguing-in-Publication Data

A catalogue record for this book is available from the British Library

ISBN 0–85969–862–9

Typeset by Deltatype Limited, Birkenhead, Merseyside
Printed in Great Britain by Biddles Ltd
www.biddles.co.uk

For my brother in medicine, Manu Tailor,
GP in Great Witley, Worcestershire

Contents

Introduction

Who would want to read a book on prostate cancer? At first thought, very few. Men who already know they have the disease, and their partners, are an obvious readership. Relatives of men who have had it, and who think they may get it themselves, are another. Yet another target group includes men who have had the odd problem with their ability to urinate and who may be wondering about their future, and are even frightened about it.

This book aims to help all these people, but it is for a much wider group than just them. It is for anyone with an interest in enjoying a healthy old age, regardless of whether or not they fear prostate cancer in particular. There are several reasons for this. Most important among them is the fact that prostate cancer has, until recently, been the 'hidden epidemic' among us. While breast, lung, and bowel cancers have hit the headlines time and again when a new treatment for them has been launched, the constant stream of good news about prostate cancer coming from the research institutes and hospitals has rarely seemed to excite the newspaper editors.

Partly that has been due to ignorance of the prostate gland and its importance. This ignorance exists just as much among many media people who write and broadcast about health matters as in the rest of society. Even some of the most prestigious newspaper, magazine, radio, and television journalists still persist in mis-spelling and mis-stating *prostate* as *prostrate*. I have had my own copy for health columns mis-corrected in this way many times by sub-editors: it makes me frustrated and angry. If people whose very job depends on their excellent knowledge of the English language get such things wrong, there is little chance that the rest of the public will be any better informed than they are.

That is sad, because in countries where huge efforts have been made to educate the public about prostate cancer, there is evidence that deaths from the disease have passed their peak and may even be declining. The hidden epidemic is no longer hidden in the United States. Better public awareness of prostate cancer there has led to earlier diagnosis and therefore to earlier and more successful treatment. Combine these pieces of good news with newer treatments that cure or give long-term relief from prostate cancers, and the war against them is beginning to be won. The American Cancer Society, using figures from the US National Cancer Institute, has shown that since the early 1990s deaths from prostate cancer have declined by around 7 per cent.

This welcome fall in deaths from prostate cancer has not been because there have been fewer cases. On the contrary, the number of cases of prostate cancer has been rising all over the developed world, the United States included. The rise is set to continue and become even steeper as the proportion of older men in each country rises further. In 1994, Drs R. and M. Kirby and Drs J. and A. Fitzpatrick predicted the increase in numbers of men over 60 years old in various countries by the year 2020. The United Kingdom's projected increase was the lowest, at 60 per cent. The figures for the United States, Japan, and Canada were 120, 160, and 210 per cent respectively. Writing now in 2001, they have been proved accurate so far.

What is the relevance of these population figures to prostate cancer? The answer is that men's risk of developing this type of cancer, more than any other, rises steeply as they grow older. This does not mean that everyone with prostate cancer is so old that there's not much point in treating them. Far from it. The rise in risk starts at age 50 to 54, with a death rate from prostate cancer of 8 per 1,000 men in the population of that age group. The figure rises to 23 by ages 55–59, 68 by 60–64, 140 by 65–69, and 260 by 70–74. In 1990 in England and Wales 12,423 men younger than 75 died from prostate cancer. This makes it number three in the causes of early death from cancer – after breast cancer in women, and lung cancer in both sexes.

So a major aim of this book is to help reduce these figures. The best way to do this is to persuade more men to seek early diagnosis of any minor symptoms related to passing urine. Only a small proportion of such symptoms turn out to be due to prostate cancer, but it is vital to sort them out from all the other, more minor, causes. That is because the earlier that prostate cancers are diagnosed, the more likely it is that they can be completely cured – for even now, by the time of diagnosis, around half of all prostate cancers have already spread outside the boundaries of the gland. By definition they cannot be completely removed at this stage. This book describes the many new treatments for this stage of cancer that prolong life and alleviate the symptoms, but *cure* for it is still some years away. It would be far better if many more prostate cancers could be 'caught' earlier, at a stage when cure is feasible. And it has to be said that the pattern of progression of most prostate cancers, which is usually slow and predictable, makes cure a real probability in most people for whom the diagnosis has been made in the earlier stages.

There is another group of men, however, whose prostate cancers can be diagnosed at an earlier stage still, when they have no symptoms at all. These are the men who, because of heredity, have a higher risk than others of developing the disease. A father, brother, or uncle has had the disease, usually at a younger age than most, say in their fifties. If they can go back further in their family tree they may find more men who have died early from the disease. There is a very strong case for them to be 'screened' for prostate disease using blood tests. Tests for detecting the earliest stages of prostate cancer are improving rapidly, and a chapter of this book has been devoted to them.

However, applying such screening for early prostate cancer to the general population with no history of the disease in the family, and no symptoms of early prostate cancer, is still controversial. It is argued, fairly, that many small prostate cancers that are found on screening will never progress in the man's expected lifetime to a stage where they will cause symptoms, far less death, from the disease itself. Finding these cancers would be a disadvantage, as it would add unnecessary stress and fear to individuals' lives. So the section of this book that deals with screening also looks at ways in which prostate cancers that are likely to be the ones that truly need treatment can be distinguished from those that can be left alone. We doctors are still not very good at making this vital distinction, but we are improving.

The first part of this book is therefore about diagnosis of prostate cancer. It is for men who have heard of it and would like to know more about it – so it should be of interest to any man in middle age and beyond. The second part is about the treatment of prostate cancer. Here most readers will be men who have had to face the diagnosis, along with their concerned partners, relatives, and friends.

This is where the good news starts. Even now, in the twenty-first century, the word 'cancer' is commonly associated with imminent death. That view is firmly dispelled by the book's section on treatment. There is optimism on all fronts among the people who wage the war on this disease. Surgeons have found better ways to remove diseased prostate glands, while preserving sexual function and feelings (a real drawback in the past). Physicians have found better drugs to slow and even arrest the spread of the disease. And there is great optimism for the future, particularly with the ever-expanding knowledge of the mechanisms by which prostate cancers are initiated and then spread within the body. Molecular biologists and geneticists are combining their knowledge to produce ways of reversing the underlying causes of prostate cancer, and these will eventually reach the clinic.

Details of the genetics and molecular biology of prostate cancer are outside the scope of this book, but it would not be complete without giving you a flavour of what is happening in these areas, because they offer such hope for the future. So my chapter on them is an optimistic one.

Men with prostate cancer can live successfully, happily, and with fulfilment. This is the book's overall message. If you or a partner, relative, or friend have the illness, then please read it. It aims to support and lighten the burden, and not to depress.

Here I must pay a debt to several doctors without whom this book could not have been written. First to Dr Jonathan Waxman, of London, with whom I worked some years ago. He guided me, and first fired my special interest in this disease. Also, my thanks go to two other Londoners, Roger Kirby and Timothy Christmas, and their colleague Michael Brawer, of Seattle. Together these three men wrote *Prostate Cancer*, the definitive book for doctors on this disease. As a general practitioner, I obviously do not have their personal experience of research and of the specialist treatments in which they are so expert. So I have had to draw on their book for many of my facts. Any reader, medical or not, who would like to know much more about prostate disease could not do better than read their book. It is beautifully written and illustrated, though it will hardly be used as a coffee table ornament!

1

The Normal Prostate Gland

Let's first make the name clear. It is the *prostate* gland, not the *prostrate*. Prostrate things lie flat – and that's nothing to do with prostate, which is derived from the ancient Greek, meaning 'to stand in front of'. The word was first applied to what we now know as the prostate gland, according to medical historians, by Herophilus, a Greek living in Alexandria around 335 BC. Herophilus was slightly out in his anatomy, because it lies beneath the bladder rather than in front of it. He can be forgiven for that small mistake, because doctors did not add to his knowledge of the gland in the following 2,000 years.

Why do we have a prostate gland? First, it provides most of the fluid that forms the ejaculate. The testes provide the sperm, which passes along tubes upwards through the groin and into the abdomen, where it collects in the seminal vesicles, small 'bags' lying just above the prostate. During ejaculation, sperm from the seminal vesicles mixes with a much larger volume of fluid from the prostate gland to form the ejaculate, or semen.

To function normally, therefore, the prostate must be made up of two main tissues. They are the glands and ducts that form and transport the fluid, and muscle fibres that provide the power to propel the fluid out of the prostate into the urethra – the tube from bladder to penis through which the ejaculate must flow during orgasm.

The prostate is therefore wrapped around the base of the bladder, surrounding the urethra. About the size and consistency of a small orange (such as a tangerine), it has the two seminal vesicles lying above and to the side of it. The ducts within the prostate lead into an opening in the urethra, as shown in Figure 1. Above the prostate lies the base of the bladder, within the walls of which are muscle and nerve fibres that are very sensitive to the pressure of urine within the bladder. Also around the side of the prostate is the network (the medical word is *plexus*) of nerves that control and co-ordinate the outflow of urine from the bladder, and also erection and ejaculation.

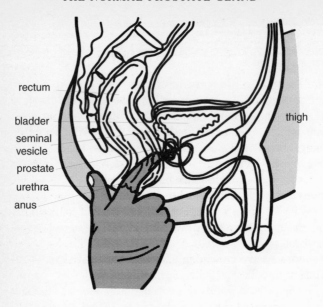

rectum

bladder

seminal
vesicle

prostate

urethra

anus

thigh

Figure 1
The prostate gland and its relationships
to bladder and nerve plexus

It is important to bear these anatomical facts in mind when trying
to understand why problems with the prostate produce such diverse
symptoms. For example, when the prostate enlarges for any reason,
it can compress the urethra. Naturally that makes it more difficult to
pass urine. Because the urine is passing through a narrower tube, you
need more force to expel it, and the flow can be slower and more
difficult to sustain or maintain.

If disease of the prostate invades upwards, it can put pressure on
the base of the bladder. That can upset bladder control, so that you
may feel you need to pass urine more often than normal
('frequency'), or the signal of needing to pass urine may be stronger
and more pressing than normal ('urgency'), or you may get feelings
of incomplete emptying of the bladder.

Invading in other directions, disease of the prostate may interfere
with the nerve plexus around it, causing impotence, or interfering
with ejaculation. It may destroy sexual feelings in the penis. And
disease within the prostate can cause internal bleeding in the organ
so that blood appears in the ejaculated sperm.

2

Of course, there are causes of all these symptoms other than prostate cancer, but any one of them should alert men to the possibility of this disease. How doctors distinguish them is dealt with in Chapter 5.

It's also important to an understanding of the prostate and how it may go wrong to know a bit about its internal structure. Our present knowledge of prostate gland architecture stems from work by Dr J. E. McNeal, who was the first to divide the prostate into three zones. The biggest is what he called the peripheral zone, which occupies most of the lower two-thirds of the gland substance. Most of the upper third of the gland is taken up with the central zone, which lies just underneath the bladder and to the rear of the urethra. Between 5 and 10 per cent of the prostate consists of the transition zone, which wraps around the upper third of the urethra, in front of the central zone and above the peripheral zone. Figure 2 shows how they all relate to each other: the urethra, the seminal vesicles, and the base of the bladder.

Front View   Side View

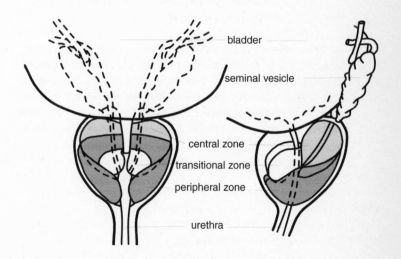

Figure 2
The three zones of the prostate and how they relate to
rectal examination

The three zones of the prostate differ subtly according to their microscopic appearance, the details of which are not relevant to this book. What is important to know about them is that when a doctor does a rectal examination of the prostate it is the peripheral zone that is in direct contact with his or her finger, and that most prostate cancers arise in this zone. In contrast, most cases of benign prostatic hypertrophy or hyperplasia (BPH), which is the main cause of prostate symptoms (BPH is far more common than prostate cancer), arise from expansion of the transition zone, which encroaches on the peripheral zone. A skilled doctor can usually tell the difference between the two, at least when the diseases are in their early stages.

It is also important to understand that all cells in the prostate, regardless of the zone they are in, produce substances called prostate-specific antigen (PSA) and prostatic acid phosphatase (PAP), about which much more is explained later in this book. They are vital to the diagnosis and to determining the progression of prostate cancer. Two more substances crucial to understanding prostate cancer are growth factors and androgens. It is enough to state here that growth factors seem to be more concentrated in the central and transition zones and androgen receptors in the peripheral zones. Knowing about this has led researchers to a new understanding of ways to combat prostate cancer.

Most prostate cancers (more than 70 per cent of them) arise in the peripheral zone, which makes them, as mentioned above, relatively easy to detect on rectal examination. However, this ease of detection is counterbalanced by the fact that they are closer to the neural plexus than tumours arising in deeper parts of the gland, and are therefore more likely to cause early sexual problems, such as impotence and failure of ejaculation. The next chapter describes in greater detail how an enlarging prostate can cause problems.

2
When the Prostate Goes Wrong – the Natural History of Prostate Cancer

Finding the cancers that may kill

It must be admitted that most men with recognized prostate cancer are beyond their middle ages: they are over 70. And in many of them, the cancer progresses very slowly, so that they can live ten years or more with their disease, and ultimately die from a quite unconnected problem, such as a heart attack or stroke. This has led to some doctors suggesting that most prostate cancers are better not found, as they only cause men to worry unnecessarily about dying from a disease that is not going to kill them.

There is good reason for this viewpoint. Post-mortem studies of men dying from other causes have found incidental small areas of cancers in their prostate glands in 20 per cent of men in their twenties, 30 per cent of men in their fifties, and in 70 per cent of men over 80 (Sheldon, Williams and Fraley, 1980, pp. 626–31). These were microscopic areas of cancer that had caused no symptoms in the men's lifetimes. If the men had survived the disease, or avoided the accident (or even act of murder) that had killed them, very few of those cancers would eventually have developed enough to have become obvious. Many of them must have been very slow-growing. A much more important statistic is that fewer than 10 per cent of men will develop symptoms of prostate cancer in their lifetimes, and fewer than 3 per cent will actually die from the disease.

What we really need is to be able to detect early those cancers that do develop, and that somehow escape the body's mechanisms that protect us against them. Happily, we are getting much better at doing just that.

Inheriting prostate cancer

The first pointer to better protection against progressive prostate cancer is that men who have had a relative with the disease have a higher than expected risk of developing it than men who have not. The fathers and brothers of 228 men with prostate cancer were three times more likely to have the disease than those of a similar number of men without prostate disease (Woolf, 1960, pp. 739–43). A large study in the Mormon community in the United States showed that prostate cancer has a stronger tendency to be inherited than bowel or breast cancer (Cannon and Bishop, 1982, p. 47). Men with two close relatives with prostate cancer have five times, and men with three close relatives with it 11 times, the lifetime risk of the illness than people with no such relatives (Steinberg, Carter, Beaty *et al.*, 1990, pp. 337–40). It is now accepted that about 9 per cent of all prostate cancers have a genetic background.

This news has two consequences. One is that all men with prostate cancer in the family should be regularly screened for the earliest signs of the disease. This should start at a relatively young age, say around 40 years, because inherited prostate cancers usually show themselves much earlier in life and are more aggressive in their behaviour than those in men with no relatives with the disease. Such cancers detected early, before symptoms start, have a near-100 per cent chance of cure by modern surgical and medical methods. These cancers are described in Chapter 10.

The other consequence is that this knowledge has stimulated much research into exactly which gene is responsible for the cancers. So far, the exact site or sites of the problem have not been identified, but it is proposed that the change that leads to the cancer is loss of, or mutation in, a gene that normally suppresses cancerous change, and that it lies either on chromosome 1 (of our 23 pairs of genes) or on the X chromosome. This is no place for a detailed description of how genetics can be manipulated to help cure cancers, but this information does offer hope, in the sense that researchers are on the way towards finding practical methods of restoring defective genes to normal.

Geography makes a difference

Another clue to the origins of prostate cancer is the wide variation between countries in their incidence of the disease. The Scandina-vians have the highest prostate cancer detection rates, at around 60 cases per 100,000 men per year. This compares with figures of 50 in the United States, 20 in the United Kingdom, and only 4 in China and Japan. Why should these figures be so different? The numbers of deaths from prostate cancer in the United States and the United Kingdom do not differ nearly so much – they are 20 per 100,000 in America and 12 per 100,000 in Britain. These figures tend to confirm that many men diagnosed as having early prostate cancer in the United States (who are exposed to strong pressures to be 'screened') would not develop obvious disease if left without treatment, and might be better left undiagnosed.

However, earlier diagnosis from better screening alone does not explain why Japanese men emigrating to California or Hawaii have more than twice the prostate cancer rate of those living in Japan (though still far less prostate cancer than Californians of European or African descent or native Hawaiians). There are similar rising figures for migrants into the United States from China and India. The common theme running through all these studies is that there is a basic incidence of prostate cancer in every community that may be increased by some environmental factor, the main one probably being diet. But there are other factors, such as levels of male sex hormone, that must be taken into consideration.

Male sex hormones

The prostate gland cannot develop to maturity without male sex hormones circulating in the blood. They are collectively known as androgens, the best known of which is testosterone. So the prostate gland remains small until puberty, when teenage boys become awash with testosterone. Along with acne and an interest in the opposite sex comes a rapidly enlarging and functioning prostate gland.

However, testosterone has its drawbacks, and one is that prostate cancer does not develop without its presence. Men who have inherited defects in sex hormone production – medically speaking, they are 'pseudohermaphrodites' – do not develop mature prostate glands, or prostate cancer. Nor do eunuchs. However, there is no direct relationship between the levels of testosterone in men's bloodstreams and their risk of prostate cancer. It is not true that the higher your testosterone level, the greater the risk you have of developing prostate cancer. In fact, it is only as men grow older, and their testosterone levels are falling with age, that the cancers start to show themselves.

One reason for this is the long 'latent period' between the first cancerous change in a prostate cell and the cancers becoming big enough to cause symptoms. Another is the fact that testosterone is not the real culprit. Inside the prostate gland testosterone is converted into a much more active hormone, dihydrotestosterone, or DHT, by the enzyme 5 alpha-reductase. This may seem a bit too technical for a book like this, but it is important to know about it, because this reaction is the basis for one of the most successful means of treating prostate cancer. DHT, and not testosterone, is now known to be the androgen that stimulates the growth of the prostate in puberty, and which is needed to keep the mature prostate working at maximum efficiency during men's sexual lives. Its downside is that it is also a powerful stimulus to prostate cancer cells to keep growing.

That is one of the many areas of new knowledge about prostate cancer in the last 20 years that offers hope for its treatment. Once researchers knew about 5 alpha-reductase and its activity in producing DHT, they were soon working on drugs to block its action, and so stop the growth of prostate cancer cells. There is now a series of drugs for prostate cancer, the 5 alpha-reductase inhibitors, that do exactly that. They are widely used not just to shrink tumours in the prostate gland itself, but also to reduce the volume of 'metastases', secondary areas of prostate cancer distant from the initial (or 'primary') site. There is more about metastases and their treatments in Chapter 15.

Evidence that 5 alpha-reductase is important in prostate cancer comes from studies of men who are born without the ability to produce it. They form one group of the pseudohermaphrodite men mentioned above: their prostate glands remain in the pre-pubertal state, and never become cancerous. Differences in inherited levels of 5 alpha-reductase may also explain, at least partly, the big variations in prostate cancer rates in different areas of the world. A 1992 *Lancet* report proposed that the lower prostate cancer rate in Japan is linked to the fact that Japanese men have, on average, much lower levels of 5 alpha-reductase than men elsewhere.

We have known for many years, too, that men with cirrhosis of the liver are much less likely than normal to develop prostate cancer. This has been linked to the finding that cirrhosis leads to lower levels of testosterone, and higher levels of the female sex hormone oestrogen, than normal in men. Both of these hormonal changes in theory should reduce any risk of developing prostate cancer.

What you eat and prostate cancer

Oestrogens are present in food, so some foods should also protect against prostate cancer. One reason behind the low incidence of prostate cancer in Japanese and Chinese men is that they eat many more root and green vegetables than men in the West. Present in such vegetables, and particularly in soya, are plant-based oestrogens ('phyto-oestrogens') called genistein and daidzein. Men who eat enough of them alter the balance of male and female sex hormones in their blood – and that change is enough to lower their risk of prostate cancer. Japanese men who have taken to Western eating habits and eat less vegetables have a higher rate of prostate cancer than those who stick to traditional Japanese diets.

Phyto-oestrogens are not the only substances in food that may influence our chances of developing prostate cancer. The high numbers of cases in the United States overall have been correlated with eating high amounts of animal fats, mainly derived from dairy products and red meats. Within the United States, the regions in which the consumption of fats and dairy products is highest are also the regions with the highest prostate cancer rates. In a strict follow-up over many years of 4,700 men working in the health professions (Giovannucci et al., 1993a, pp. 1571–9), 300 developed prostate cancer during the study. They had eaten significantly more red meat than those who had no prostate disease. The link was strongest among Americans of Asian descent.

Why should eating fats increase prostate cancer risk? One possible cause, taken from animal studies, suggests that they speed up the change from normal cells to cancer cells in a prostate influenced by testosterone levels. Another is that eating high amounts of animal fats reduces our ability to absorb vitamin A. This reduces the blood levels of beta-carotene, the active form of the vitamin, which some studies suggest helps prevent prostate cancer developing. Vegetables are high in vitamin A, and when men change to a vegetarian low-fat diet their blood testosterone levels fall by 30 per cent (Hill and Wynder, 1979, pp. 273–82). This should also lower the chances of developing testosterone-stimulated prostate cancer.

On the whole, therefore, people with eating habits that include mainly foods high in animal fats and that are low in varieties and amounts of vegetables must face the fact that they are raising their risks of prostate cancer.

And the evidence strongly suggests that the way to lower that risk is to eat better, rather than just to take vitamin or mineral supplements. Several studies in which vitamin E (alpha-tocopherol) or vitamin A (beta-carotene) were added to the normal eating habits of men have produced mixed, even startling, results. Alpha-tocopherol supplements, for example, have been reported to reduce prostate cancer rates, but only in smokers. Yet prostate cancer is one of the few cancers not definitively linked to smoking. Beta-carotene supplements have actually been linked to increases in prostate cancer in two separate studies, one in the United States (Heinonen *et al.*, 1998, pp. 440–6), and one in Scandinavia (Tretli *et al.*, 1996, p. 128).

One group of researchers has stressed that prostate cancer cases increase the further the men live from the equator, and suggest that it may be due to vitamin D deficiency (Schwartz and Hulka, 1990, pp. 1307–12). (Vitamin D levels are lower, generally, in people who are exposed to less overhead sunshine. The skin makes the vitamin from sunlight.) In the laboratory, adding vitamin D to cultures of prostate cancer cells prevents them from becoming cancerous and multiplying out of control (Feldman *et al.*, 1996, pp. 53–63). However, studies of human populations with different vitamin D levels in their blood have not produced clear conclusions that it prevents either the initiation or the spread of prostate cancer.

No link with sexual activity?

Because the prostate is an organ whose only function is connected with the sex act, it has been assumed that prostate cancer is linked to excessive sexual activity. Proposed links to cancer have been made with an earlier than normal start to one's sex life, multiple sexual partners, perhaps a past episode or episodes of sexually transmitted diseases, and a high frequency over many years of sexual intercourse. The last is difficult to judge, as there is too little information from enough men to know what is a higher frequency than normal.

Suffice it to state here that although one study proposes a link between prostate cancer and gonorrhoea caught about 45 years before, another has related increases in prostate cancer rates to lower than normal sexual activity in men. Possibly the bravest study on this subject was on deaths from prostate cancer in 1,400 Catholic priests. It must be assumed that this group of men, all of them avowedly celibate, had had much less sexual experience than the rest of the male population! The conclusion was that they had just the same death rate from prostate cancer as other men.

So it is difficult to draw any conclusions on whether sexual activity increases or decreases the risk of prostate cancer, or whether it makes no difference. If having sex earlier, and having more sexual partners, both make a difference to prostate cancer rates, then we will find out soon, because the age of first intercourse for British men has dropped to 17 years, from 20 years a generation ago. And a *Lancet* review reported that the numbers of sexual partners men have in a lifetime has increased steeply over the same years (*Lancet*, 1994, pp. 899–900).

Other influences on prostate cancer

In 1994, Chinese doctors reported that prostate cancers were more common in cities than in country districts, and that city dwellers were more likely than countrymen to die from them (Gu *et al.*, 1994, pp. 688–91). They suggested that industrial pollution might provoke prostate cancer. They listed workers exposed to chemicals in the rubber, textile, chemicals, drugs, fertilizer, and atomic energy industries as being at high risk of prostate cancer. Which chemicals may be the direct cause they did not know, but one chemical high on the suspect list is cadmium. The atomic energy industry in Britain has been seeking connections between prostate cancer and radioactive forms of hydrogen, chromium, iron, cobalt, and zinc. So far, none have been proven.

Could prostate cancer be the result of a viral infection? Viruses are known to 'trigger' the development of other cancers, including cervical cancer in women, so it is feasible for viruses to do the same in men. The difficulty has been in identifying possible virus candidates from prostate cancer material. A typical study reported antibodies to herpes simplex virus type 2 (well known to the public as 'genital herpes', and linked to cervical cancer in women) in the blood of 71 per cent of men with prostate cancer and 66 per cent of men with benign prostate hyperplasia (BPH). The detection in blood of antibodies to a virus indicates a past infection with the virus. Herpes virus has been detected in prostate cancer cells, and one study – not, as far as I know, confirmed by any other – suggests that wives of men with prostate cancer are themselves at higher than usual risk of cancer of the cervix.

For the moment, the jury is out on whether viruses may cause prostate cancer. If eventually they are found to do so, this leaves the way open to exciting new treatments: but antiviral drugs for prostate cancer are still a long way off.

Vasectomy and prostate cancer

Probably the most contentious issue on prostate cancer is whether or not it may be caused by a previous vasectomy, perhaps many years before. In 1990, Drs L. Rosenberg and J. R. Palmer and their colleagues (1990, pp. 1051–9) suggested that the operation may lead to cancerous change in the prostate. Their work was heavily criticized for technical reasons. Some support for them appeared in 1993 with two studies by Dr E. Giovannucci and colleagues. One looked into past results, and one followed a group of men into the future until they did, or did not, develop prostate cancer (Giovannucci et al., 1993b, pp. 873–914). Both groups showed a slightly increased rate of prostate cancer among the men who had had vasectomies. Much larger studies, however, did not find such a link (Sidney, 1987, pp. 795–7; and Stanford et al., 1999, pp. 881–6).

These conflicting results leave doctors like myself in a quandary. Many couples ask for advice on vasectomy. It is widely held to be safe and harmless. The evidence suggests that there may be a very small risk that it may cause prostate cancer in a few men. Or there may be no risk at all. I tend to tell men considering whether to go ahead with vasectomy that a future small risk of prostate cancer is a possibility. If the man has no close relative who has been affected by the disease, I tend to leave him to discuss it with his partner: most go ahead with the vasectomy. A man who is already at higher risk (because of a father or brother with the disease) often asks for guidance. I tend to advise against vasectomy in his case, for two reasons. One is that we do not know if there is an added risk in such men, and it seems foolish to take the chance. The second is that if he eventually develops prostate cancer after a vasectomy, he will feel guilty and blame himself for submitting to the operation. That is no mental attitude with which to fight the disease.

BPH and prostate cancer – are they related?

Another common question asked of doctors is from men who already know they have BPH (benign prostatic hyperplasia). It is: Will my BPH turn into prostate cancer? Here, as with vasectomy, the researchers have come to different conclusions. At first sight, a link between the two is unlikely. The two diseases arise mostly in two different zones of the prostate: cancer in the peripheral zone, BPH in the transition zone. In 1974, however, N. K. Armenian and

12

colleagues reported that men with BPH subsequently develop prostate cancer three times more often than men with apparently normal prostate glands. This report was countered by P. Greenwald and colleagues, who found a reduced risk of prostate cancer in men with BPH (Armenian *et al.*, 1974, pp. 115–17; Greenwald *et al.*, 1974, pp. 35–40).

The fact is that both BPH and prostate cancer are common in older men, so that by chance it is likely that both diseases will coexist in many men, without the first having developed into the second. I see no need to add to the existing worries of men with BPH by suggesting that they need extra tests to rule out cancer, or that they must be extra vigilant, because they are at higher than normal risk of developing it. The evidence suggests that they are not.

How the cancer will progress – if it does

The next most common questions about prostate cancer are asked by men when they first hear that they have it. How is it going to develop? Am I going to die soon? It is difficult to answer them, because nowadays treatments are very successful. Surgery, radio-therapy, and drug treatments all alter the course of the disease and may eradicate it altogether. But what about leaving the cancer alone, and letting it follow its natural course?

That sounds stupid and cruel – but it may not be. In 1994 G.W. Chodak and his colleagues collected and analysed the results of letting the disease take its natural course, with no medical or surgical intervention, in 828 men whose prostate cancers were confined to the gland itself (Chodak *et al.*, 1994a, pp. 242–8). It would be impossible to repeat their research today, as there is too much pressure upon the doctors to treat every prostate cancer actively, with surgery, radiotherapy, or medical treatment. Yet many doctors like myself wonder, after the Chodak group's results, whether some men with prostate cancer would not be far better untreated.

The Chodak report showed that 94 per cent of the men whose cancers were, on microscopic appearance, 'well-differentiated' survived for at least ten years after their diagnosis. This was in contrast to only 58 per cent of the men whose tumours were classified as 'poorly differentiated'. A 94 per cent survival for another ten years in men of their age is virtually normal, so it is reasonable to conclude that treating these men would not have

13

offered them any advantage over just 'waiting and seeing' how they got on.

The crucial point about the Chodak findings is the phrase 'well-differentiated'. This means that the cancer cells seen under the microscope still look like prostate cells. They are clearly cancerous, but they are not the fast-multiplying 'undifferentiated' cells that will produce a rapidly growing tumour. They may be so slow growing that they will never enlarge enough to cause pressure on the bladder, the urethra, the nerve plexus around the prostate, or invade into the blood vessels around it. In effect, men with this type of tumour will probably never have serious problems with it. They may even be the men whose tumours would have been detected in their twenties, and that have never developed beyond the microscopic state.

The 'poorly differentiated' tumour carries with it a different outlook. The cells of this type of tumour look much less like their parent normal prostate cell. Instead they are a mass of cells with no obvious normal prostate tissue among them. They have much more dense centres: in a single 'field' under the microscope there will be several cells that are obviously dividing – splitting into daughter cells. They are the cancers that will spread, form obvious masses within and outside the prostate, and eventually lead to early death. They must be treated aggressively with all that the cancer team can throw at them.

This knowledge leaves doctors in a dilemma. It is easy to deal with the 'poorly differentiated' type of cancer – there is no doubt that it has to be treated and eradicated if possible. But what should be done about the 'well-differentiated' types? A small minority of them will become more aggressive if left to themselves. The problem is how to predict which ones will do so. The various tests in which 'prostate markers' are used to try to do this are explained in Chapter 7, but it must be admitted that they are not perfectly reliable. So, in practice, everyone with a diagnosis of prostate cancer is now treated, so as to ensure that those cancers that will change to a more malignant phase will be dealt with.

The stages of prostate cancer

There are three main steps in the development of aggressive prostate cancer. The earliest is the appearance of microscopic clusters of cancer cells within the prostate gland: clusters that produce no symptoms and cannot be detected by normal physical examination. The second phase is for these cells to grow in bulk within the prostate gland to a size that is detectable by physical examination and is starting to cause symptoms, such as urinary problems. In the third phase, the cancer spreads outside the prostate gland into the tissues immediately surrounding it, such as lymph glands in the pelvis and abdomen, and then distantly into bones, such as spinal vertebrae.

How this progression occurs is still a matter of fairly heated argument among the experts. One group believes that all prostate cancers eventually follow this route from stage 1 to stage 3 in time (Stamey, 1982, pp. 67–74). Some cancers are simply slower than others in doing so. They have evidence that it can take four years for a prostate cancer to double in size, so that it may be ten years before it reaches 1 ml in volume. This is the size at which many cancers start to cause symptoms, although many more are undetected until they are two or three times as big.

Other researchers propose that for prostate cancers to progress they need to undergo several successive genetic mutations (Carter *et al.*, 1990, pp. 742–6). The first mutation may produce the well-differentiated cancers mentioned above, but they need a second to turn them into aggressive undifferentiated cancers, and perhaps a third to cause them to spread further than the prostate. The chances of men having three successive mutations in a cancer are very small, which is why aggressive, life-threatening cancers are relatively rare. This could be why so many men with microscopic cancers never go on to have serious disease.

This 'multistep' explanation for the development of cancer may also explain why, although microscopic prostate cancer rates are similar all over the world, the rates of aggressive, spreading cancers differ widely. In the countries with the higher prostate cancer death rates, environmental conditions that lead to mutations may be changing the nature of the disease.

How these mutations can happen is explained in more detail in the next chapter. By necessity it is complex, so if you wish you can skip it, and turn to Chapter 4, which describes the ways in which prostate cancers show themselves. However, if you wish to know the latest thinking on how prostate cancer arises and develops further, then Chapter 3 is a must for you.

3

The Science behind Prostate Cancer

The prostate gland has a very complex architecture. It comprises glandular cells producing fluid of very intensely controlled composition (its components must be kept within extremely well-defined limits to be of maximum benefit for the sperm); ducts collecting the fluid; muscle cells that expel the fluid from the ducts; fibres that supply the 'skeleton' for the gland; nerves to co-ordinate the function of all these elements; and blood vessels to supply oxygen and nutrients.

None of these structures are static. The cells within them are constantly dying off and being renewed. They are continually exposed to hormones and 'growth factors' that stimulate their growth, and to the effects of genes that initiate their 'suicide' when they are too 'old' to function normally or are showing signs of becoming cancerous. It is when the balance between growth and death of cells is disturbed that prostate cancers start. This brief chapter summarizes the latest thoughts and knowledge about how that disturbance can occur.

The foremost influence on prostate cell growth are male sex hormones. To the general public, the best known of these is testosterone. The word is in public use as a synonym for male strength and sexual potency. Testosterone itself is made in the testes and, as mentioned earlier, without it the prostate cannot develop. However, the testes are not the only source of male sex hormones. A small amount (much less than formed in the testes) is made by the adrenal glands, which lie over the upper surface of the kidneys. They produce two 'androgens' – hormones like testosterone that stimulate male sexual function – called androstene and androstenedione.

In normal circumstances, the effect of adrenal androgens on the prostate is tiny, as they are overwhelmed by the effects of testosterone. But if all testosterone is removed, such as by castration, or by drugs that block the effect of testosterone, then the adrenal androgens will still continue to stimulate prostate growth. This effect is vital when it comes to treating prostate cancer – it is sometimes necessary to remove the effect of adrenal, as well as testicular, male sex hormones from the prostate cancer cells. How this is done is explained in more detail in the chapter on treatment of prostate cancer.

It must be added here, for the sake of completeness, that the effects of testosterone and adrenal androgens on the prostate are not straightforward. To stimulate prostate cell growth they must first be converted, within the prostate, into dihydrotestosterone (DHT). This is done by a substance also produced in the prostate, called 5 alpha-reductase, or 5 alpha-R. If the action of 5 alpha-R can be blocked, then the prostate cells, normal or cancerous, lose the biggest stimulus to their growth. Without 5 alpha-R, the cell suicide pathway is unopposed. Within ten days of starting treatment to block 5 alpha-R, 90 per cent of the prostate cells are undergoing 'suicide' (Bruchovsky *et al.*, 1975, pp. 61–102).

This is why one of the first attacks on prostate cancer – or, for that matter, benign prostate overgrowth or hypertrophy (BPH) – for many men is a drug to block 5 alpha-R. But it is not the only chink in the prostate cancer-cell armoury.

New genetic techniques have identified genes in the prostate that stimulate the cell suicide process. Genes are usually given a three-letter identity and sometimes a number, and convention dictates that they are printed in italics. The 'good' genes, as far as prostate cancer is concerned, in that they promote cancer cell suicide, are *bax* and *bcl-2*. Another family of genes needed for control of normal cell growth is called *Cdc2*: they work along with a protein called cyclin to help prostate cells grow in an orderly, non-cancerous fashion.

These genes do this by forming substances called 'growth factors' (GFs). This is not the place to explain in detail how growth factors stimulate cells to grow and multiply. It is enough here to list the growth factors that have been identified in prostate tissue – they include epidermal GF, insulin-like GF, fibroblast GF, and transforming GF, among several others. Named mainly after the tissue or system that they stimulate, they are vital to understanding future treatments of prostate cancer. If the GF that stimulated the growth of a particular cancer can be identified, and its effects neutralized, or can be removed from the equation, then that cancer will stop growing. Research to achieve this aim is well on the path to success.

So how do prostate cancers start, and then continue? Knowledge of hormones, genes, and growth factors has given us many clues. Cancer of any tissue starts when a mutation, or several mutations, occur inside a cell that gives it an advantage in growth (or in resisting the message to commit suicide) over the cells surrounding it. No longer responding to the normal controls, it starts to produce 'daughter' cells by dividing in two. (Cells divide in order to multiply, a curious anomaly for the mathematical mind.) As the numbers of its descendants increase, there is an increasing chance that one of them will undergo a further mutation, and the cancer will become less like the original normal cell. In medical terms, it becomes 'de-differentiated'. This process eventually leads to the cells developing an ability to spread through the surface of the prostate to the surrounding tissues in the pelvis, and then, by breaking into blood vessels, being carried in the circulation to distant sites in the body, where they can lodge and grow. This is called metastasis.

This series of cancer-inducing steps takes time, which is why most prostate cancers do not make themselves obvious until later middle age or old age. But it is common in the longer run: the experts predict that around 9 per cent of all men develop prostate cancer in their lifetimes. Thankfully, only a small minority of them, however, go on to die from their cancers.

Why do some men get them, and not others? For the answer we must go back to those genes. Some men possess 'oncogenes', genes that with a single mutation can alter the balance between growth and suicide in prostate cells. Many have already been identified. They include genes labelled as *ras*, *sis*, *c-erb*, *c-myc*, *c-fos* and *c-jun*. When these genes go wrong, they constantly give the cells the signal to grow and multiply and to ignore the suicide call. However, the body has its own way of protecting itself against oncogenes. It also possesses 'anti-oncogenes' or 'tumour suppressor' genes that oppose the activity of the oncogenes.

For example, one anti-oncogene was found by Professor David Lane and his team at Dundee University. Called *p53*, it stimulates cell suicide when it detects any abnormality inside the cell that may suggest a pre-cancerous change. If *p53* is absent or bears a mutation that stops this vital function, the person has a highly increased risk of cancer, including prostate cancer. One research group found changes in the *p53* gene in up to 80 per cent of prostate cancer specimens (de Vere White *et al.*, 1993, p. 376A).

Stimulation of cell growth is only the first step. For the cancer to spread outside the prostate it needs also to be able to break through the surface, known as the 'capsule'. For that to happen, other genetic mutations have to occur. The cancer cells have to lose the natural tendency of prostate cells to stick together inside the architecture of the organ. Cells normally stick together by means of 'cell-adhesion' molecules, called E-cadherin. The gene that forms E-cadherin is known to be sited on chromosome 16 (we have 23 pairs of chromosomes plus the sex chromosomes XX or XY). If that gene fails, then cells easily burst through the prostate capsule to spread within the pelvis.

Once outside the prostate, the cancer cells need to have a blood supply to stay alive. Amazingly, the researchers know how they form their own new source of blood. Cancer cells secrete substances (they are called angiogenesis factors) that stimulate the growth of new blood vessels around them, so that they can survive and grow elsewhere in the body. There is even an 'antimetastatic factor' identified on chromosome 17, produced by gene *nm23*, that acts against the angiogenesis factors. When that is lost, the cancer can spread beyond control.

All this new scientific information may seem frightening to anyone with prostate cancer or caring for someone with the disease. It is not meant to frighten, but to reassure – because the more we know about the mechanisms that cause cancer first to develop, then to spread within the pelvis, and finally to distant sites in the body, the better we are able to fight it. Already this knowledge has led to the development of drugs to block 5 alpha-R. They have had spectacular results in the clinic. Our knowledge of genes and chromosomes is leading to the identification of oncogenes, so that men at high risk can be watched to ensure that even the earliest change can be caught and dealt with as soon as it arises. New ways of identifying prostate cancer 'markers', substances that signal changes in chemistry before tumours are large enough to cause symptoms, have been developed. One marker, prostate specific antigen, is already being used routinely to identify cancers and to follow progress of treatment. It has a chapter to itself in this book.

Although gene therapy is a few years away yet, there is progress towards ways of blocking oncogenes, renewing failed anti-onco-genes and tumour suppressor genes, and we are close to ways of improving people's own immune system responses to prostate cancer.

We are already using androgen suppressor drugs to slow down and even arrest prostate cancers. We are drawing ever closer to finding medicines that will suppress the other growth factors that stimulate cancer cell growth, and to blocking angiogenesis. So there is optimism in the air among prostate cancer researchers and specialists. I hope this book can spread similar optimism among men with the disease too.

4

Some Case Histories

My first case history comes from 30 years ago, in the early 1970s. It is here only to show how much our treatment of prostate cancer has improved over the last few decades. Please don't let it frighten you, as it is not what happens today.

James was 62 when he went to his doctor for the first time. He had not the slightest suspicion that he had anything wrong with his prostate gland. His main problem was pain low down in the centre of his back. It was there all the time, a persistent ache that never left him. It didn't matter what he was doing, bore no relation to the time of day, often kept him awake at night, and was neither worsened nor relieved by opening his bowel or his bladder. He didn't look well, was rather thinner than his doctor remembered from a year or two before, and admitted to vague tiredness and general lack of energy. He was shocked, when his doctor weighed him, to find he had lost nearly 10 kg (a stone and a half). He thought that he had lost a little weight, but not that much.

This combination of loss of weight and persistent pain sounded ominous to his doctor, who decided to subject him to a thorough physical examination, a series of blood tests and some X-rays. The diagnosis became apparent on the rectal examination. The doctor's finger came up against a firm non-tender swelling in the lower part of the prostate, quite discrete from the rest of the gland, which was smoother and softer to the touch. He was immediately referred to the local urology clinic, where after a further internal examination he was put on the only treatment then available: the female hormone oestrogen.

James's pain and feeling of ill health improved very quickly. He was less tired and was able to return to work. But he had severe side effects. He lost his sexual drive, his chest began to change shape so that he had feminine breasts that became embarrassing to him, and he lost his facial hair. He no longer had to shave, but he did not look on this as an advantage. Instead, he felt he was no longer a man. These side effects were tolerable because he knew the alternative, worsening bone pain, was even worse. James survived eight years before the cancer symptoms 'broke through' the oestrogen therapy. He then rapidly worsened, and died.

Now, 30 years later, men like James can look forward to a much better quality of life with their treatment for prostate cancer. Take Ian, the second case history, as a comparison:

Ian's first visit to his doctor was in April 2001. All his life he had been a successful, physically very active, farmer, and still walked over his fields and hill every day to check the stock. So when he started to feel a bit breathless and tired after only half a day's stroll, he thought something must be wrong. His only other symptom was a persistent headache that did not respond easily to aspirin, and a difficulty in moving his right hip. He could not flex it up against his abdomen as easily as he could move his left thigh. His doctor confirmed that there was some restriction of movement of his right thigh, but not his left one.

His doctor, who was also an old friend, was struck by his pale appearance and the fact that he had lost some weight. So he took the symptoms seriously and arranged blood tests and an electrocardiogram (ECG). Ian turned out to be anaemic – his haemoglobin was around 12 g, instead of the usual 15 g. There was nothing specific about the other blood tests, and his ECG was normal. But because he had not had a thorough check-up for some years, his doctor performed a rectal examination. The prostate was enlarged and had a firm, craggy 'feel', and was larger on the right than on the left side. It seemed a bit 'stuck' against the surrounding tissues, and was not as easily moved about in the pelvis as a normal gland would be.

His doctor immediately sent him to the local hospital urological department, where the diagnosis of prostate cancer was confirmed. A 'prostate specific antigen' (PSA) test was done, and a bone scan ordered. Happily, in this part of Britain, it was arranged within a week. The PSA turned out to be as high as 550 units, strongly suggestive that the cancer had spread beyond the confines of the prostate gland. He did not have to wait for treatment. It was started on the day he saw the consultant – a three-week course of cyproterone acetate pills, with an injection every three months (started a week after the first cyproterone pill) of Zoladex. Within a few days he was feeling much better, and he should be able to look forward to many years of active life in good health.

Why Ian was given this treatment, the significance of the PSA test, and the need for the scan are explained in Chapter 5. It suffices for the moment to use his case as an illustration of one way in which the illness is diagnosed.

Unfortunately, both Ian's and James's cases are, in reality, failures. Their prostate cancers were diagnosed too late for them to be cured, for their cancers to be eradicated altogether. Until around 1980, this was the way the vast majority of men found they had the disease. They came to their doctors only after they were losing weight, had pain in their bones, were tired all the time, had little energy, and trouble passing or retaining urine. Treatments of advanced cancers like this have improved hugely over the years, but they still do not eradicate the disease completely. They often stave off death from prostate cancer until the men who have them die from something else, like a heart attack or stroke, or even 'old age', but the cancers remain in a relatively dormant state. There is always the possibility that they will become active and cause serious disease.

Happily, since the early 1980s we have become much better able to detect prostate cancers in their early stages, before they have spread, and that gives us the chance to remove them completely with new types of treatments and operations. The last half of this book is devoted to how we can do this now, and even improve in the future.

So my third case history is about one of these more 'modern' men, Frank:

Frank's discovery that he might have prostate cancer came out of the blue. Called by his doctor for a 'well man' review on his fifty-fifth birthday, Frank was sure that he would be given a clean bill of health. He was fit and enjoying a successful life at the top of his career, and looking forward to some time with his wife now that the children were grown up and away from home.

One routine 'well man' test is a rectal examination. A finger gently inserted into the anus will detect abnormalities in the lower part of the bowel and the prostate. Frank did not find it uncomfortable or even unpleasant, but he was shocked to hear his doctor say that he might have a problem with his prostate. The finger had felt a small lump, harder than the rest of the prostate, near the lower surface of the gland. His doctor explained that further blood tests would have to be performed, including a PSA test, and that he must see the local urologist, who had a special interest in prostate disease.

Events passed very quickly from then on. He saw the urologist that afternoon. He confirmed that it was probably a prostate cancer. The PSA measurement suggested that it was still localized to the gland itself, as did the ultrasound examination (see Chapter 8 for details). For the first time in his life, Frank became concerned about his health. His doctors explained that there were two choices for him. One was to do nothing, and have repeated checks every six months or so of the size of the tumour, the PSA level, and also of his general health. He was not anaemic, and blood tests showed no problem with any other organs. A whole body scan to detect possible metastases was negative.

It came as a shock to Frank that he could have cancer yet his doctor could suggest that he might not need treatment. There was logic in this advice though. Many prostate cancers are very slow growing and cause no problems for years. Treating them may be more of a bother to their 'owners' than waiting for them to become more active. That can take years.

The alternative for Frank was to remove the prostate gland in a 'radical prostatectomy', an operation that would remove the whole gland and with it the possibility of life-threatening disease (see page 57). After a discussion with the consultant surgeon, and particularly because he was relatively young, Frank decided to go ahead with surgery. It was highly successful: Frank no longer needs to fear his prostate, and his PSA has dropped to the very minimum.

Tony, in his sixties, like Frank had his prostate cancer diagnosed by chance. His doctor had taken part in a trial to see if screening for cancer in the general population was worthwhile. Part of that screening was a routine PSA blood test. Tony's turned out to be well above normal – too high to ignore. Yet his prostate gland felt normal to the rectal examination. The ultrasound test showed no real change in the gland's make-up, and there was no obvious site from which a biopsy (removal of a piece of the gland for examination) could be taken. Tony's consultant was adamant about his management. He advised no treatment for the moment, and only to take steps if there was any change when Tony returned for follow-up over the next few months.

It wasn't easy for Tony to accept this policy of 'wait and see', but when it was explained that most prostate cancers were slow growing and any change would almost certainly be detected before it would threaten his life, he became reconciled to it. Now, two years later, with no rise in his PSA and no obvious cancer developing, he is happy that he decided not to undergo surgery, with its discomfort and problems.

Tony's cancer was found on routine screening. Screening for prostate cancer in the general population is still controversial – unlike screening for breast cancer in women which, in 2001, was proven beyond all shadow of doubt to have brought down the deaths from breast cancer by around 60 per cent in most developed countries. This is a huge forward step in cancer detection and management, and if screening for prostate cancer could do the same for men, it would be at least as beneficial, if not more so. So Chapter 6 is about prostate screening, who should have it, and how it is done.

Before going on to screening in detail, however, it is best to clarify the symptoms that men may develop if they have prostate disease, and how they may mean either BPH or prostate cancer.

5

Explaining the Symptoms

Symptoms of prostate disease – do they indicate cancer or benign hyperplasia (BPH)?

First, and most important, any man over 45 years old who is concerned that he may have prostate cancer should be given the opportunity to be screened for it. He may have no symptoms at all, but just wish to make sure that he is not at risk. A father, uncle, or brother may have had the disease, or he may just have a friend or colleague with it, and wish to reassure himself. If he sees his doctor, he will have two very quick tests – a rectal examination and a PSA test (using blood from a forearm vein). If the two together are negative, he can be reassured, and worry no more. A five-yearly re-examination is probably adequate from then on.

It is different if there are symptoms that indicate that prostate cancer is possible. To understand how they may arise, think back to Chapter 1, which describes where the prostate gland is, and its relationship to the bladder and its outlet tube, the urethra. A tumour (growing mass) inside the prostate can compress the urethra and interfere with the delicate nerve and muscle mechanisms at the base of the bladder – and in doing so may hinder the fast and strong flow of urine from the bladder to the penis. As the tumour grows larger, it can extend beyond the normal boundaries of the prostate gland, invading other structures within the pelvis. For example, it can grow into the bladder itself, to cause blood in the urine, or it can compress the ureter, the tube from the kidney to the bladder, causing pain running from the loin (in the small of the back) to the groin.

Then small parts of the tumour can break away from it, to be deposited in distant parts of the body, such as the bones of the spine and pelvis. This can lead to back pain, anaemia, tiredness, and listlessness, along with weight loss, as the active cancer deposits (they are called metastases) use up vital energy stores.

Experts in prostate cancer therefore divide the symptoms of prostate disease into three groups – those of bladder outflow obstruction, those caused by local extension of the tumour into the surrounding pelvic tissues, and those of distant spread.

Bladder outflow symptoms

There are seven main symptoms of bladder outflow problems. They are:

- poor stream of urine;
- hesitancy (difficulty in starting to pass urine);
- sensation of incomplete emptying after passing urine;
- intermittency (stopping and starting during urination);
- frequency (having to pass urine more often than before – but not necessarily more urine at a time);
- urgency (having to pass urine urgently because of a sudden need that is hard to control);
- and urge incontinence (wetting yourself because you have not been able to reach the toilet in time).

It must be said here that none of these symptoms are exclusive to prostate cancer. Most are common with BPH (explained in Chapter 1). Some are caused by a condition called irritable bladder, in which the nervous system that the bladder uses to detect that it is becoming full is too sensitive, and makes you feel that it is full when it is still half empty. But if you have these symptoms, you must have your prostate checked, as you cannot ignore them.

They are so well recognized that the American Urologic Association has established an 'International Prostate Symptom Score' (IPSS) which has been endorsed by the World Health Organization for use in diagnosis and in clinical trials. IPSS is an excellent way to measure the severity of any urinary obstruction and bladder floor irritation in prostate cancer, and to assess the response to treatments. IPSS is fully explained here, so you can use it yourself and judge your own progress for yourself. Bear in mind that you should give each of the first six questions a score from 0 to 5:

- 0 = Not at all
- 1 = Less than 1 time in 5
- 2 = Less than half the time
- 3 = About half the time
- 4 = More than half the time
- 5 = Almost always

The questions all relate to how you have been in the last month:

1 *Incomplete emptying*: How often have you had a sensation of not emptying your bladder completely after you finish urination?

2 *Frequency*: How often have you had to urinate again less than two hours after you finished urinating?

3 *Intermittency*: How often have you found you stopped and started again several times when you urinated?

4 *Urgency*: How often have you found it difficult to postpone urination?

5 *Weak stream*: How often have you had a weak urinary flow or stream?

6 *Straining*: How often have you had to push or strain to start urinating?

Question 7 is scored slightly differently. It is:

7 Over the last month, how many times did you most typically get up to urinate from the time you went to bed at night to the time you got up in the morning? This time, the reply must be chosen from the following:

- 0 = none
- 1 = once
- 2 = twice
- 3 = 3 times
- 4 = 4 times
- 5 = 5 times or more

The final question is on your quality of life. If you were to spend the rest of your life with your urinary condition the way it is now, how would you feel about that? Score it as follows:

- 0 = delighted
- 1 = pleased
- 2 = mostly satisfied
- 3 = mixed – about equally satisfied and dissatisfied
- 4 = mostly dissatisfied
- 5 = unhappy
- 6 = terrible

You will see that you can score from 0 (no problems at all) to 35 (worst of all) on the symptoms score, and from 0 to 6 on the quality of life score. On the symptom score, 0 to 7 is considered mild, 8 to

19 moderate, and 20 to 35 severe. Repeat scoring over the months after the start of treatment can give researchers (and, for that matter, yourself) a good idea of how well you are responding to treatment, and how effective the treatment is. It has the extra advantage that the numbers can be used by statisticians to evaluate results in large-scale trials of new treatments.

The quality of life score, which remains separate from the symptom score, is mostly used as a basis for discussion between patient and doctor about management of the illness and how to improve it. A good quality of life score, for example, influences the decision on whether or not your doctor contemplates surgery or other radical treatments, or whether to leave well alone until the quality of life deteriorates.

Although the International Prostate Symptom Score is useful, it does not help to differentiate prostate cancer from BPH. Because so many men have BPH, most men with prostate cancer also have some degree of BPH, and the outflow symptoms are more likely to be caused by the BPH than the cancer itself. As mentioned in Chapter 1, BPH usually arises in the transition zone close to the urethra, and is therefore more likely to put pressure on the urinary outflow than cancers, which usually arise much more commonly in the peripheral zone, further from the urethra. This is why some men have 'distant' symptoms of prostate cancer without ever having had any trouble with urine flow.

So, unless the tumour has started in the transition zone, or has become very large, early symptoms of bladder outflow problems are more likely to be due to BPH than to cancer. One way to help differentiate between the two diseases is to divide the bladder outflow symptoms into two types: obstructive and irritative.

Obstructive symptoms, which are caused by the enlarging mass pressing on the urethra, include reduced flow, hesitancy, and incomplete emptying. They are more likely to be due to cancer than to BPH (although they can be caused by either). The ultimate obstruction is urinary retention, in which urine flow stops, the bladder over-fills, and the patient has a distended abdomen and severe pain. The harder he tries to expel urine, the worse it gets. The only answer is to pass a catheter (a sterile hollow flexible tube) up through the penis past the obstruction, or through the front of the lower abdomen (suprapubic catheterization), to empty the bladder.

Irritative symptoms include frequency and urgency. They are the result of the expanding mass in the prostate pressing up against the base of the bladder, interfering with the delicate 'detrusor' muscle system that co-ordinates and controls the emptying of the bladder as it begins to stretch with a full load of urine. The detrusor system is the one that gives you the message that your bladder is needing to empty. You can ignore it for a while, but it returns with its message as the need becomes more urgent. A mass just below the detrusor stretches it, fooling it into believing that the bladder is fuller than it is. Hence the frequency and urgency. Irritative symptoms are more common with BPH than with prostate cancer, but, like obstructive symptoms, both conditions can cause them.

Bladder outflow symptoms can lead to complications beyond the prostate. For example, a 'pool' of urine left in the bladder after incomplete emptying can easily become infected: it is a perfect place for germs such as bacteria to multiply. This can lead to pain in the bladder (which you feel in the lower half of the abdomen, between the navel and the pelvis), much more frequency and urgency, and pain passing urine (this is 'dysuria'). Such infections may lead to obvious blood in the urine. If you pass blood in the urine it is just as likely to be due to infection as to a bleeding tumour, so do not assume the worst. But do report it to your doctor.

This static pool of urine in the bladder is also a perfect medium in which 'stones' can form. These are made of particles of calcium or crystals of a waste substance called urate. Also called 'calculi', they can irritate the bladder, again producing pain just above the pelvis, and blood in the urine, especially as the act of urination is finishing. Germs find it easy to grow on their surface, so they can also cause urinary infections. Sometimes the first sign of prostate cancer or BPH is the discovery of a stone in the bladder during a straightforward X-ray for pain in the lower abdomen. Any man who is found on X-ray to have such a stone must have his prostate fully investigated. How this is done is explained in Chapter 9.

Symptoms of local spread

All the symptoms described above relate to men whose tumours have not progressed beyond the boundaries of the prostate gland itself. However, they do overlap a little with the symptoms of the next stage of the disease – spread within the pelvis beyond the prostate. Prostate cancer specialists list nine symptoms typical of prostate cancer that has spread beyond the gland itself, but is still confined within the pelvis. They are:

- blood in the urine (haematuria);
- pain passing urine (dysuria);
- general lower abdominal pain not linked to passing urine;
- impotence;
- incontinence;
- pain in the loin (the angle between the lowest rib and the spine in the back);
- signs of back pressure of urine on the kidneys;
- severe constipation and bleeding from the rectum;
- blood in the sperm (haemospermia).

The blood in the urine in this case comes not from a bladder infection, but from direct invasion of the tumour into the urethra. The incontinence arises from the tumour invading the 'sphincter' (the muscle at the base of the bladder that closes off to stop the flow of urine into the urethra). The pain may come from acid urine running over a raw cancer surface in the urethra. Impotence happens if the tumour invades the complex nerve, blood vessel, and muscle structures that lead to erection. Extension of the prostate tumour upwards can block urine flow from the kidneys into the bladder, leading to back pressure on the kidneys, and hence the loin pain. As this blockage becomes more severe, the back pressure can damage the kidneys, leading to their eventual failure. And backwards extension of a prostate tumour may lead to pressure on the bowel, which lies just behind it. Some prostate cancers are found in the clinic for rectal disorders, because their only symptoms are of bleeding (it is common for haemorrhoids to be blamed) or a change in the normal bowel habit towards severe constipation.

This sounds a horrific list of symptoms, but it is very rare indeed for any one man to have them all. They are presented here so that you can understand why you have your particular set of symptoms, and to reassure you that they can all be tackled with the correct treatment. Once you know why a symptom has arisen, you are well on the way to devising a solution to it. And that is what all prostate tumour management aims for. How we find out what is happening in each individual case is explained in Chapter 9.

Of course, all of these individual symptoms may arise because of other illnesses. Impotence, for example, is a common accompaniment of diabetes in some older men. It may result from stress, or be a side effect of drugs prescribed, for example, for high blood pressure. The important message here is, if you have one or more of these symptoms, to let your doctors know about them, and to be willing to undergo extensive questioning and tests to find out their cause.

Symptoms of more distant spread

Unfortunately, more than half of all men with prostate cancer already show spread of their disease beyond the prostate into the pelvis, and a quarter show spread to distant sites, such as bones, at the time of their diagnosis. This limits the options for treatment and cure: if these cases could have been detected earlier they might have been suitable for a more comprehensive attack on their tumours. The only way to do this in the future will be by accurate screening for early prostate cancers, the pros and cons of which are discussed at length in Chapter 8.

The symptoms of more distant spread – metastases – arise both from the site at which the cancer cells have lodged and from the general malaise that they cause. How they affect men with them is listed here, the first six being signs of metastases at a particular site, the last three being their effects on general health:

- bone pain;
- spontaneous fractures (breaks) of bones;
- weakness, numbness, or paralysis of a leg;
- enlarged glands in the groin or elsewhere;
- swelling of the legs;
- pain in the loin;
- lethargy and listlessness;
- weight loss;
- bleeding from skin and bowel.

Bones, in particular, are the sites of metastases, so they often cause pain in a rib, or the pelvis, or a long bone, such as in the arm or leg. However, the most common pain of distant spread from prostate cancer is in the spine in the back. The start of pain low in the back that does not ease with rest is a fundamental sign of prostate cancer that has spread beyond the pelvis. Sometimes the invasion of prostate cancer cells into the bones can make them vulnerable to fractures, especially if you bear weight upon them. A broken hip in an elderly man who may have had some urinary outflow problems must be considered a case of prostate cancer unless proved otherwise.

Pain in the back due to prostate cancer deposits in spinal bones can lead, if untreated, to collapse of the relevant vertebra, and this in turn can put pressure on the nerves that run into the spinal cord above and below the collapse, and on the spinal cord itself. This 'spinal cord compression', in which there is pain or numbness and weakness – leading even to paralysis – in the legs, can even be the very first sign of prostate cancer in some men. Any sign of persistent unusual back pain in an older man, especially if there is weakness or numbness, must be treated as an emergency. Removing the activity of the cancer cells (by 'androgen deprivation', by radiotherapy, or surgery – see Chapter 15) can lead to dramatic improvement in the pain and other symptoms, and can prevent paralysis.

Extension of the tumour into the bone marrow, where the blood is produced, interferes with the production of new red blood cells, leading to anaemia. Cancer cells spread along 'lymph channels' via the groin and alongside the main vein from the abdomen to the heart, the vena cava. Lymph glands (much like the tonsils in the throat) that are stationed along the lymph channels react to the cancer cells with an 'immune response', so that they swell and become much firmer. They become most noticeable, of course, when they are near the skin, and that means, for spread from the prostate, glands in the groin are usually the first to show the problem. They become obviously enlarged and very firm, but are not necessarily painful.

Normally these lymph glands in the groin are on the lymph drainage path from the legs back into the body. Lymph is the fluid in which all our tissues are bathed. It constantly flows in lymph channels from the tissues to the centre of the body, where it eventually empties into the main veins to the heart. At regular intervals along the lymph channels are lymph nodes or glands that contain masses of white cells called lymphocytes. They act as protectors and filters against inflammation and infection, and also against cancer cells. Cancer cells that enter the lymph system meet up with the lymphocytes in the lymph nodes, where they cause inflammatory reactions that lead to the swellings that are noticed, initially, in the groin.

In this fight to the death between the cancer cells and the lymphocytes, the flow of lymph from the legs may be blocked within the enlarged glands, and lymph builds up in the leg beneath. This leads to a swollen leg, the swelling extending from groin to foot, the medical name for which is lymphoedema.

Men with this stage of the disease usually also show, on specialized X-ray or ultrasound examinations, similarly enlarged glands along the line of the vena cava to the right of the spine inside the abdomen. Some of them may be so large that they press upon the ureter from the kidney on that side – and that can cause back pressure upon it, leading to a persistent dull ache in the loin. Later in the spread, if it is not checked, swollen glands may appear as far from the prostate gland as the armpit or neck.

The relevance of spread of your cancer

Why is it so important to know if your cancer has spread, and to which sites? In the past, a diagnosis of metastatic prostate cancer was disastrous. There was little to be done to stop a steady progression to terminal illness and death from the disease. Now, we have many ways in which we can arrest the disease, and the treatment and long-term management depends on an accurate diagnosis not just that the cancer exists, but also of where it is, its extent, and its susceptibility to each of the treatments we can use against it. So if you have been told your cancer has spread, it is no longer a death sentence. It is a challenge for both you and your doctors, but it is one that is very worthwhile taking up. Writing in 2001, and as a practising family doctor in a rural area of south-west Scotland, I know of at least four men who were given the diagnosis of metastatic prostate cancer before 1990, and who are still well. One is now 69 and still easily outplays me at golf. There is every reason for you, if you have been given the same diagnosis, to try to emulate these men. Your doctors will surely help you in doing just that.

Their first task in doing so is to find out how extensive your prostate cancer is: in effect, they will 'stage' your tumour. How that is done is the subject of the next chapter.

6

Staging and Assessing Your Tumour

We 'stage' prostate cancers in different ways. The doctors' first task is simply to perform the routine examination of the abdomen that they learned as students, and have perfected with experience. That involves looking for lumps in the groin, 'tapping' (percussing one finger against another lying flat on the abdominal surface) for an over-full bladder, looking at the legs for swelling, then placing a finger in the rectum.

The rectal examination is still the best way for the experienced doctor to assess the prostate. In the United Kingdom it is done with the man lying on his left side, the knees drawn up to the chest. In the United States, it is usually performed with the man standing, and leaning forward against a wall. Some doctors now employ a knee-elbow position, on the grounds that it gives a better 'feel' of the whole prostate gland. As most tumours arise in the peripheral zone, i.e. the part of the gland that is nearest the finger, rectal examination is remarkably accurate in detecting cancers.

The earliest stage that can be detected is a firm 'nodule' like a hard pea, that is well within the gland, not altering its shape. This is defined as stage T2a or B1, depending on the system used by the clinic. Stage T1 is a cancer usually found almost by accident, during tests for BPH, with no indication of tumour on rectal examination. It is described below in the paragraph on 'TURP'.

Stage T2b or B2 cancers feel harder still and are larger and more diffuse, with a less well-defined edge, but remain localized to one side of the gland. Stage T3 (or C) cancers are larger still, and distort the normal prostate outline, but the gland remains mobile and unfixed to the surrounding tissues. Stage T4 (D) cancers lead to hard, misshapen, enlarged prostates that are much less mobile because they are fixed to the surrounding pelvic structures. They are the cancers most likely to be linked to distant metastases.

Experienced family doctors and all specialists in prostate gland disease can usually tell the difference between cancers and BPH by the 'feel' of the prostate surface and its texture. BPH feels softer and has more 'give' in it than cancer, and the swelling of the gland is much more symmetrical than cancerous masses. However, there are other prostate conditions that are more easily confused with cancer.

One is chronic prostatitis.

Chronic prostatitis is the result of recurrent infections ('acute prostatitis') in the prostate gland. These bouts of acute prostatitis are fairly easy to diagnose. They involve all the usual signs of infection, such as fevers, sweating, and pain in the lower abdomen. The acute illness also causes severe pain on passing urine, sometimes with blood in the urine, and can be mistaken for a urinary infection. However, the give-away sign is a very tender, but soft, prostate on rectal examination. Doctors have to be very careful doing rectal examinations in men with acute prostatitis, as it can elicit extremely severe pain.

The treatment for acute prostatitis is the appropriate antibiotic, but in some cases the infection lingers on. That can eventually lead to hard deposits of calcium (sometimes giving a gritty feeling, or even presenting like a prostate 'stone') that may feel like a cancer. Chronic prostatitis often accompanies BPH, so that the gland is enlarged too, making confusion with cancer even more likely.

Most of the time the rectal examination alone is enough to confirm or rule out prostate cancer, but there are cases when it is impossible to differentiate between chronic prostatitis and prostate cancer. This is one reason for all suspected cases to be subjected to biopsy – a piece of the prostate is removed and examined under the microscope.

Biopsy

Experts in prostate diagnosis can use their finger in the rectal examination to guide a fine needle into the gland. Biopsy needles are made so that they can take a piece of material (the biopsy) from the precise site of the abnormality. However, doing it using the finger only is not always easy, so that most biopsies are now taken under the guidance of an ultrasound scan. An ultrasound probe is inserted into the rectum, and an automatic device removes the biopsy during the scan. This is called Trans Rectum Ultra Sound, or TRUS for short. In most prostate units today every suspicious area of prostate is subjected to TRUS biopsy. In fact, TRUS biopsies are also performed in men who have been found at screening (perhaps because of a high PSA – see Chapter 7) to be at high risk of prostate cancer, even if there are no suspicious areas on rectal examination. TRUS may find early lesions that cannot be felt by even the most experienced finger.

TURP

Sometimes the diagnosis of prostate cancer is made incidentally after surgery for BPH. Some men with bladder outflow symptoms (see Chapter 5) have, on rectal examination, obvious BPH, and there is no sign of prostate cancer on rectal examination. They are then offered 'trans-urethral resection of the prostate', or TURP for short.

The best way to describe TURP in layman's language is that the enlarged piece of prostate around the urethra (in the transition zone – see Chapter 1) is 'bored out' by passing a flexible instrument up the urethra into the region of the prostate. It then rotates, and cutting blades are used to remove, in slices or 'chippings', the overgrown prostate tissue that is causing the obstruction. The pieces of tissue that are removed during TURP are collected and viewed under a microscope for any signs of malignancy.

A 1991 report (Altwein *et al.*, 1991) found that as many as 10 to 20 per cent of men undergoing TURP for apparently benign prostate disease actually had traces of cancer in their TURP chippings. These are the stage T1 (or A) cancers described above. They are divided into T1a (A1) and T1b (A2). In T1a disease the tumour cells have a less malignant appearance and occupy less than 5 per cent of the chippings. In T1b disease, more than 5 per cent of the chippings show cancerous changes, and they look more malignant.

Why stage?

Why should we bother to stage prostate cancers, and what can we do with the information? Staging is crucial to the decision on how, or even whether, to proceed with treatment. There is no need for me to remind readers that for a man to be told he has prostate cancer is devastating – although this is not always the case. I've known men be grateful for at last knowing what was wrong, after months of feeling generally unwell. Even though they had to face up to the fact they had cancer, it was better than not knowing. Now that they had a tangible enemy to fight, they felt better. And they felt better still when they started their treatment, and the activity of their cancers began to wane, almost instantaneously.

Not every man needs treating. In men over 75, the staging process may indicate that the cancer is unlikely to spread quickly or to cause serious problems for many years. They may not need any active treatment, but a follow-up examination every year or so, to make sure things have not changed for the worse, and that treatment need not yet be started. For men younger than 75, who could fairly be expected to live at least another five years, accurate staging and appropriate treatment may help to prevent their disease from developing further and from metastasizing. Staging can identify the men who will benefit most from the different forms of treatment that can now be offered to them. They are described in the last part of this book.

However, before we turn to treatments, we need first to understand the subject of 'tumour markers' and how their level in the blood affects how we treat and follow up men with prostate cancer. The one we use today is prostate specific antigen, but more are to come.

7

Prostate Specific Antigen (PSA) – and Future Tumour Markers

If there was one thing doctors would like to have for every cancer it is a 'tumour marker'. This is a simple blood test that shows us how active a cancer is, even when the patient is still feeling well and has no symptoms. It is then that the disease can be treated before it causes symptoms, and may even be kept under complete control. So we are fortunate in that the best tumour marker of all is found in prostate cancer. It is prostate specific antigen, or PSA.

Technically speaking, PSA is a glycoprotein, a compound of protein and sugar, that is formed only by the cells in the lining of the prostatic ducts, the tiny tubes that carry the prostatic fluid to the urethra. Its normal function in the body is to break down proteins formed in the seminal vesicles, small sacs at the back of the prostate in which sperm from the testicles collects. Although most PSA remains within the prostate, some 'spills over' into the bloodstream. PSA levels in prostatic fluid, for example, are one million times higher than those in the blood, but still this 'spill-over' PSA can be measured, very accurately, in blood taken from a vein.

There were early problems devising an 'assay' (a method for measuring PSA), but the newest methods are extremely reliable. Higher than normal blood PSA levels occur in prostate cancer, and not in any other form of cancer. In most men with no prostate disease, the PSA is less than 4 nanograms per millilitre (ng/ml). The figures do rise with age, but even in extreme old age, in men without prostate cancer, PSA levels are hardly ever above 10 ng/ml in most laboratory assay systems.

PSA levels also rise, and stay high for two weeks, after needle biopsies of the prostate are taken, after TURP (see page 37), and even after catheters and other instruments are passed into the urethra. They are therefore usually measured either before your surgeon performs any of these procedures, or at least a fortnight afterwards.

Moderate rises in PSA (to around 20 ng/ml) may be recorded in men with BPH or prostatitis, and in the early stages (T1a and b) of prostate cancer, but the bigger rises, of 50 to 800 ng/ml, are found in more advanced cancers (stage T4). The main reason for a steep rise in PSA, therefore, is active prostate cancer. This is why PSA measurement was originally approved in the United States and Europe, including Britain, for use in following the progress of men with known prostate cancer. More recently its use has been extended to early cancer detection and screening.

PSA levels relate quite closely to the stage of the cancer. Doctors from Stanford University Hospital in California have shown that each gram of prostate cancer tissue adds 3.5 ng/ml to the blood PSA level (Partin *et al.*, 1990, pp. 747–52). Values above 10 ng/ml usually mean that the cancer has spread beyond the limits of the normal gland. However, this does not necessarily mean distant metastases. The Mayo Clinic prostate cancer group reported that only one of 306 men with proven prostate cancer and PSA levels below 20 ng/ml at initial diagnosis had positive bone scans for metastatic cancer.

PSA is therefore valuable in the initial diagnosis, in that it reflects how much active cancer there is, and whether it may have spread. It is also extremely helpful in judging how well treatment has worked. For example, within a few weeks of starting successful treatment, PSA values should fall steeply, towards near-zero. Most men with undetectable PSA levels after, for example, a radical prostatectomy (surgery to remove the whole prostate in men with no spread beyond the gland itself – see Chapter 11) remain disease-free permanently. They can be considered cured of their cancers. In the few whose PSA subsequently rises again, this is the first sign of a recurrence of their disease, and it indicates that further treatment may need to be initiated to prevent spread.

However, in one report of 230 men followed for four years after this form of surgery, only 41 eventually showed a rise in PSA (Stein *et al.*, 1992, p. 942). Eighty-two per cent of them survived another five years, and 72 per cent survived ten years after the PSA rise. These are good figures – for men who were mostly already elderly when they underwent their operations. They show that a rising PSA is not necessarily a death sentence: it may show that some cancer remains, but that it is not aggressive enough even to cause symptoms, far less threaten life. This is something to remember if you are told that your PSA has risen a little.

The aim of radical prostatectomy is to remove all the cancer in the prostate at one operation. It is done only in men whose cancer is thought to be confined to the gland itself, and has not spread beyond its edges either into the pelvis or into distant sites. So it is always done in the hope of a complete cure. The figures above suggest that it often fulfils that hope. When the cancers have spread beyond the prostate, either locally or distantly, then radical prostatectomy is not an option. Surgery can no longer clear the disease, and would only spread it further. So the next choice is between radiation therapy (radiotherapy) and hormonal (anti-androgen) therapy. These are described in Chapter 15. They may not offer cure, but they can arrest the progress of the disease – and the PSA measurement helps to confirm whether or not they have done so.

Radiotherapy is usually offered to men whose disease may have spread so far locally in the pelvis that its complete surgical removal is impossible. There is plenty of evidence that PSA levels fall dramatically after successful radiotherapy. In 1989, the Stanford group published the results of following men after radiotherapy: 82 per cent of them showed a significant reduction in PSA over the next year (Kabalin et al., 1989, p. 326). This is now a long time ago: progress in radiation techniques since then must have improved upon these figures. Other groups have shown that men whose PSA levels drop steeply after radiation do very well for many years afterwards. The converse is that a PSA that does not fall, or starts to rise after radiation therapy, tends to suggest persistent cancer – and that has to be treated. The usual alternative is 'anti-hormone', or anti-androgen treatment.

Anti-androgen treatment is usually offered to men who, at the time of diagnosis of their cancer, already have evidence of distant, metastatic spread (see Chapter 5). It is also used either along with, or after, radiotherapy, particularly if PSA levels have not fallen enough to rule out remaining active disease. A fall in PSA to levels near the norm (preferably under 10 ng/ml, and even better to under 1 ng/ml) is a good sign of response to anti-androgen therapy. In one study of 48 men with metastases from prostate cancer, those whose PSA levels fell below 4.0 ng/ml had a much longer period free of recurrence than those whose PSAs remained high (Miller et al., 1992, p. 956). This study also showed that a rise in PSA could be noted an average of seven months before any new symptoms arose, giving doctors and the men themselves time to prepare for further treatments.

To summarize, PSA is invaluable in diagnosing prostate cancer, in helping to 'stage' the disease, and in monitoring the results of treatment. You will continue to need repeat tests for the rest of your life. This may sound daunting, and even frightening, as you may always be fearful of it rising again, and about what may happen if it does. But for most men it is reassuring, because each time they hear that it has stayed at its normal level, they can be happy that their disease is no longer active. That means a lot.

One use of PSA, however, needs a special chapter of its own. In the United States, it is used to 'screen' apparently healthy men for the earliest stages of prostate cancer. Should this practice be adopted elsewhere? On the surface, it would seem to be of great benefit, but the concept of screening for cancer is still a matter for debate. If you are reading this book because someone close to you has prostate cancer, and you are worried that you may yourself develop it, then you may have thought about being screened for prostate cancer. Please read the next chapter before you do so. It puts forward the current arguments for and against screening. There are pros and cons about discovering that you have an early prostate cancer.

8

Screening for Prostate Cancer

I have to say here that I am in favour of cancer screening. I am sure as a doctor that if I have patients, male or female, who are in the early stages of a cancer that has not yet grown large enough to cause the symptoms that would bring it to their notice, I would like to know about it. It is a general rule that the earlier we can detect a cancer, the greater the chance we have of curing it completely.

This is certainly true of breast cancer in women. Writing in 2001, we have had breast cancer screening in Western Europe for around 30 years. For most of that time, arguments raged about whether it was useful. Did inviting all women aged 45 and older to have mammograms really reduce deaths from breast cancer? The answer was a long time coming, but it was worth it when it did. As is often the case in medicine, the Scandinavians came up with the proof. Since they started breast cancer screening, breast cancer deaths among the women who came for screening have dropped to less than half of those in women who did not attend. The drop in deaths was a staggering 63 per cent. The difference was not because women who came for screening had fewer cancers; it was because the cancers were caught so early that they were much more likely to be cured.

I would argue that the same could be done for prostate cancer, but that the benefits, if they exist, will not be shown for many years – perhaps 15 or more. That is no reason not to start now. However, in trying to be unbiased about the question of screening for prostate cancer, the two sides of the argument are laid out below.

First we must define screening. It is a process whereby doctors or other members of the primary health care team (often nurses) invite apparently well people to have a health check. The people chosen for the invitation are taken from the medical list, are usually from a particular age group, and have not had a recent examination for the problem to be screened. The aim is to find, if possible, signs of serious disease before it becomes obvious because symptoms have appeared. Simple examples are checks for high blood pressure or for diabetes, which only involve a cuff around the arm or a urine test. They are relatively cheap, and can lead to worthwhile health benefits as both can be treated very satisfactorily.

Breast cancer screening is more complex, because it involves

43

mammography. This entails an X-ray of each breast. It can often be very painful, as the breast must be compressed for the X-ray between two plates, but most women tolerate it in order to be assured that their breasts are healthy. Mammography is now proved to be more accurate than self-examination for breast lumps: it detects lumps that are too small to be detected by the woman's own hands. The big advantage in finding such small breast cancers is that we now know that there is a big advantage in doing so: treated so early, they are much less likely to lead to the woman's early death.

Screening for prostate cancer is more complex. First of all it involves a digital rectal examination. This is not pleasant. Coupled with the fact that men are more reluctant than women to go to their doctors when they are well, the thought of a rectal examination is a powerful disincentive to them to accept their doctors' invitations for a health check. PSA is also part of the screen: some men just do not wish to know whether or not they may have cancer. The thought of such an accurate blood test frightens them, and they avoid it.

However, the third reason against screening comes from some of my colleagues. They feel that making the diagnosis of prostate cancer too early simply complicates men's lives without offering them any advantages. Most cases of prostate cancer, they argue, will grow so slowly that they will never need treatment. So why give such a serious diagnosis to someone who really does not need to know? They believe that it is cruel and unnecessary, and they do have a point.

My problem with that argument is that it does not take into account the men whose prostate cancers will need treatment if we are to save their lives. Is it ethical to ignore them because we are trying not to upset the others whose cancers are not going to kill them?

The fact remains that if we wait to detect prostate cancers in men until they develop symptoms such as bladder outflow problems, or back pain due to their spread, we are consigning many of them to years of ill health. Without screening, fewer than one in three men are candidates for cure at the moment of their diagnosis, and only one in ten has such minimal and slowly growing cancer that it does not need treatment. This leaves a majority for whom treatment aims to arrest, rather than to cure, the cancer process.

With properly organized screening, we should be able to identify many more men at much earlier stages of their cancers, when we can do something radical about them. We should at the same time try to decrease the numbers of cases and to improve the effectiveness of prostate cancer treatment.

Reducing the numbers of cases may not be so far-fetched. Although we do not know why men develop prostate cancer, we do know that the drug finasteride (it is one of a group of drugs called 5 alpha-reductase inhibitors) will shrink the swollen tissues of prostate glands affected by BPH, and it is now the standard treatment of BPH. Some researchers have proposed that it may also prevent the initial stages of prostate cancer, and a large-scale trial of finasteride in the possible prevention of prostate cancer is now under way in the United States. Unfortunately it will not give results until after 2007 or 2008 at the earliest. It is hoped that wide use of this drug in men with BPH will eventually lower their prostate cancer rates.

As for improving the treatment of prostate cancer once it is diagnosed, this may be more difficult. Put simply, we have radical prostatectomy for cancers confined to the prostate, radiation therapy for cancers that have spread a little more widely, and anti-hormone treatment for cancers that have spread to distant sites. They are described in detail in the next three chapters. All are effective treatments, and even if they do not cure the cancers outright they often keep them at bay for years. However, the researchers are constantly seeking still more effective treatments, and the most promising of them are described in Chapter 18.

So if we already have reasonably successful treatments for prostate cancer, and it is a relatively common disease, why do we not screen for it much more widely? The answer lies in some unique characteristics of prostate cancer. It is alone among cancers of any organ in that it is far more common than could ever be imagined from the numbers of men in whom it causes symptoms. When prostate glands are examined at post-mortem examination of men who have died from other causes, very many more of them than could be expected contain areas of cancer. For example, in 1985, 86,000 American men were diagnosed as having prostate cancer. This was only around 1 per cent of the 8 million men in whom prostate cancers, quite unexpectedly, were found at post-mortem examination in the same year (Scardino, 1989, p. 635).

It was worked out that the risk of developing this form of 'autopsy cancer', as it was called in the United States, during an average man's lifetime was as high as 42 per cent. This was in contrast to a lifetime risk of developing 'clinical prostate cancer' (one that causes symptoms and illness) of 9 per cent, and a lifetime risk of dying from such a prostate cancer of only 2.9 per cent. Put another way, only 3 men in 1,000 with areas of cancer in their prostates actually die from the disease.

If screening for prostate cancer detects all of these cases, then what should be done with this knowledge? Treating them all with anti-cancer therapy would be like taking a sledgehammer to crack a nut, a form of 'overkill' in which far too many men would be treated unnecessarily to save the lives of a small minority. And treatment for prostate cancer does have unwanted effects (see Chapters 11 to 15 for their details).

So if screening is to be effective, it should detect only those cancers that will progress to produce illness and perhaps death, and leave undetected those that will remain low-key and unthreatening. This is not easy. We have to produce a system that detects the cancers before they cause the first symptoms, but they must only be those that we consider will cause those symptoms in the near future. By the time they have caused symptoms, the disease is often already past the stage of possible cure, and this is no longer 'screening'.

Can this be done satisfactorily with the methods we have at our disposal today? To some extent, yes. We have three screening methods: digital rectal examination (use of the doctor's finger, or DRE), rectal ultrasound, and PSA (see Chapter 7). Probably the best review of the effectiveness of these methods in detecting early cancers that need treatment is by Dr Michael K. Brawer, of Seattle, one of the authors of the best doctors' book on prostate cancer, *Prostate Cancer* (Kirby, Christmas and Brawer, 2001).

The Seattle team reported that neither DRE nor rectal ultrasound were particularly accurate, taken on their own, in detecting early cancers. Ultrasound was the more effective of the two, but it is too costly and not accurate enough to detect early cancers in a mass screening of an apparently healthy population of men. Nevertheless, the team agrees that trans-rectal ultrasound that uses a spring-loaded needle to take biopsies from a suspicious area within the prostate is the most accurate way to make the diagnosis.

PSA on its own, too, is less accurate in detecting early prostate cancer than was hoped. One problem, for example, is where to put the dividing line between a normal PSA and one that indicates abnormal prostate activity that might be cancer. In screening studies defining PSA levels above 4 ng/ml as abnormal, and below 4 ng/ml as a sign that the prostate was normal, about 2 per cent were in the abnormal range. Around one-third of this 2 per cent turned out, on further examination using an ultrasound guided biopsy needle, to have prostate cancer. So using PSA alone will detect just under one cancer case in 100 healthy men screened. Whether all the cases detected in this way should be treated is still a matter for debate.

Dr Brawer's Seattle team went further. They took PSA tests from an initial number of 1,249 apparently healthy men over the age of 50 for three years. Their aim was to see what happened to the men in whom the PSA was rising, year by year. Each year they asked the men whose PSA levels had increased by 20 per cent over the previous year's result to have a biopsy of their prostates. They reasoned that an annual increase of 20 per cent in PSA was a reliable sign that there may be an actively growing cancer. Other studies had shown that PSA in men with prostate cancer doubles every four to five years (Schmid *et al.*, 1993, p. 2031).

Using this method of a steadily increasing PSA each year, the Seattle group detected prostate cancer in around 2 per cent of their original group each year. In actual numbers, 14 men in the first year, 12 in the second year, and 13 in the third year had prostate cancers that needed curative treatment. This must be considered a good result for these men, whose future quality of life must have been greatly improved by their good fortune in having their cancers detected so early. However, Dr Brawer warns that a significant proportion (perhaps as high as one in six) of men with prostate cancers have PSA levels under 4 ng/ml at the time of diagnosis.

He mentions another worry. In the past, many prostate cancers were found incidentally when the men were having surgery (TURP – see page 37) for BPH. Their cancers were only discovered when the 'chippings' from their TURP were examined under the microscope. This opportunity for discovering cancer early is being diminished because many fewer cases of BPH are now being treated by TURP. Instead, the routine is to give them the drug finasteride mentioned above, to 'shrink' the enlarged gland, before considering TURP. Is this medical innovation, much welcomed by doctors and patients alike because it avoids or at least postpones the need for surgery, going to leave some early cancers undetected until they have spread?

This does seem possible, because the Seattle group found that 13 per cent of 91 men waiting for TURP because of symptoms of bladder outlet obstruction, and who were thought to have only BPH, were found also to have prostate cancer with real potential for causing serious illness. Admittedly they all had an asymmetrical enlarged prostate or a PSA above 4 ng/ml. These figures are a lesson for doctors to be aware of the possibility of cancer in every man thought to have BPH. All men with BPH should be screened, using rectal ultrasound (with biopsy where appropriate) and PSA, for prostate cancer.

To summarize the usefulness of screening for prostate cancer:

- Doctors are improving their DRE, rectal ultrasound, and biopsy techniques for detecting early prostate cancer.
- PSA measurements are more accurate, and a 'cut-off' point of 4 ng/ml is a reasonable one above which one should investigate for cancer.
- Repeated PSA tests that show a rise, year on year, are suggestive of active cancer.
- DRE and PSA together are very reliable in detecting early cancers that will probably cause severe disease.

The results of doctors like the Seattle team with regard to screening have led in the United States to it becoming almost as common as breast screening. It may only be coincidence, but since screening started there, numbers of prostate cancer deaths among Americans have fallen for the first time. Authors in both the Mayo Clinic in Minnesota (Drachenberg and Brawer, 2000) and in Stanford, California (Stamey *et al.*, 1998, p. 2412) write of a big shift from cases of T3 disease to T1 disease at diagnosis. This is a shift from incurable to curable cancers – and is a very welcome sign that the screening programme may already be bringing results.

Problems with screening

However, it is one thing to diagnose prostate cancer earlier, but quite another to show that by doing so, it leads to more effective treatment, saving lives and improving the quality of life. There are many reports of untreated men with known prostate cancer whose cancers never progressed to their final stages: as already stated, some older men with prostate cancer are better left untreated. That has to be balanced, though, against the 3 per cent of men who do eventually die from their prostate cancers, and who must at one stage have had early curable disease. Had they been treated in time, their deaths might have been avoided.

Large-scale trials are already running with the aim of solving this problem. In Scandinavia, the Swedish Oncology Group (oncology is the study of cancer) is randomly allocating newly diagnosed cases of early prostate cancer to radical prostatectomy (extensive surgical removal of the prostate) or to 'watchful waiting' – i.e. not treating them at all. In Denmark there is a similar trial in which men are being allocated to radiation therapy (they use a technique called external beam radiation) and what is called 'expectant management' – i.e. doing nothing until or unless an emergency arises. In the United States the PIVOT trial (it stands for Prostatectomy Versus Observation for clinically localized carcinoma of the prostate) will compare surgery with no treatment in 1,050 American men. However, we must wait for several years before we have their results, and many men, understandably, do not wish to be included in the 'no-treatment' group.

One large trial of screening for prostate cancer has already been reported, in Quebec, by Dr F. Labrie and his colleagues. They followed 38,056 men who had not been screened and 8,137 men who were screened for prostate cancer from 1988 onwards. By 1999 there had been 137 prostate cancer deaths in the unscreened group and only five among the screened men. They concluded that screening (they used DRE and PSA) followed by early treatment had resulted in a dramatic decrease in deaths from prostate cancer. Other researchers have criticized the Quebec work, because some men in each group 'crossed over'. That is, some men who were initially intended for screening were not, and some intended not to be screened were – and when the mathematics was re-worked, the decrease in prostate cancer deaths due to screening appeared to be much less. Nevertheless, considerable benefit still seemed to accrue from screening in this trial, even taking into account the cross-over numbers. A similar trial, the European Randomized Study of Screening for Prostate Cancer (ERSPC), is under way in Europe: it will be reported after 2005.

Trials are one thing, ordinary medical practice quite another. Who should do the screening for prostate cancer? Central to screening must be the general practitioners – the family doctors. Given that most men with prostate cancer are getting on in years, and that many may have other illnesses that may shorten their expectation of life, it may not be in their interest to have a prostate cancer diagnosed. As a rule of thumb, most doctors would not screen men for prostate cancer if their life expectancy, because of another illness or their age, was less than ten years.

However, family doctors who wish to screen the older men on

their lists will do so very effectively by performing a digital rectal examination and taking blood for PSA measurement. If either is suggestive of prostate cancer, then a trans-rectal biopsy will be taken from suspicious sites within the prostate gland using an ultrasound-guided instrument. The screen can be repeated every two or three years. It is done at shorter intervals if the PSA is slightly raised, and is tending to rise further on repeated sampling.

9

Investigating Prostate Cancer

Once a prostate cancer is suspected (from rectal examination and PSA), it needs to be confirmed. That is usually done by needle biopsy (a small piece of tissue removed through a hollow needle) under the view of an ultrasound probe placed in the rectum. The tissue is then examined under a microscope and the pattern of the cancer cells is assessed for their potential for slow or fast growth – that is, the cancer's potential to remain as a slow-growing tumour inside the prostate, or to become more aggressive and spread outside the gland and into distant tissues such as bone.

This assessment is called the Gleason score. Its intricacies are beyond the scope of this book, but put simply, much depends on whether the tumour cells retain their gland-like appearance and whether they retain well-defined borders (in which case the cancer will be less malign), or whether they become a mass of similar-looking cells with no hint of glands or ducts, which signifies intense malignancy. Gleason scores range from 1 to 10. Their importance is illustrated by the 1994 report of Dr G. W. Chodak and colleagues (Chodak *et al.*, 1994b, p. 242) that listed the chance of a tumour with a Gleason score of between 2 and 4 causing metastases in the following year as 2.1 per cent per year. This rose with scores of between 5 and 7, to 5.4 per cent, and with Gleason scores of between 8 and 10, to 13.5 per cent. Most men with prostate cancer turn out to have Gleason scores of between 5 and 7.

When the three main ways of assessing prostate cancers (rectal examination, PSA, and Gleason score) are put together, they become very accurate not only in staging the cancer at diagnosis, but also in helping to predict the long-term outcome, whether it is necessary to treat it at all, or how to treat it once the decision to treat has been made.

Newer tests to try to refine these predictions further are also outside the remit of this book, because they are not yet routine even in hospitals that specialize in prostate cancer treatment. They are mentioned here, however, to show that progress is being made. One is the assessment of the numbers of new blood vessels within and around the tumour. They correlate to some extent with the ability of the tumour to spread. Another technique looks for tumour cells expressing abnormal genes found only in cancer: this is still a long way from being in regular use.

Trans-rectal ultrasound (TRUS) was mentioned in Chapter 6. The newest TRUS machines will spot problems (the echo of sound returning from tumours differs from the echo received from normal tissues) as small as 0.2 mm in diameter. They can differentiate between normal and abnormal prostate tissues, and show the parts of the gland that are over-endowed with blood vessels. This last indicates either areas of active cancer or areas of inflammation due to prostatitis (see page 36).

Some prostate cancer centres are adding magnetic resonance imaging (MRI) to their investigations. MRI uses differences in magnetic fields, rather than X-rays or sound waves, to produce its images, which are remarkably clear. So far, however, comparisons with TRUS have not shown it to be any more accurate in defining the extent of prostate tumours inside or outside the gland, and it is far more expensive.

Computer tomography (CT scanning) is not helpful in assessing disease within the prostate because, unlike TRUS or MRI, it cannot reveal details of differences in texture or density of tissue inside the gland. It can detect, however, enlarged lymph glands outside the prostate, in the pelvis, and higher in the abdomen. Some centres use it when men have PSA levels above 20 ng/ml, and a Gleason score of more than 7, to see if there is spread into lymph nodes outside the pelvis. If it has spread into the lymph nodes, then this makes a difference to the decision on whether or not to operate. If CT scans do identify enlarged lymph nodes, then they may be 'dissected out' at surgery. If the affected lymph nodes are too extensive for complete dissection, then radiation therapy or anti-hormone therapy will be considered instead.

To make the investigation complete, the bones may be 'scanned' for metastases. This is done using 'radionuclides', traces of radioactive elements that are selectively taken up by cancer cells and show as 'hot spots' in the skeleton, usually in the spine and long bones of the arms and legs. Radionuclide scans are not always necessary. More than half of all men with newly diagnosed prostate cancer have PSA levels under 10 ng/ml. There is such a small chance that their tumours have spread into bone that radionuclide scanning is no longer thought to be necessary. For example, in one series of 852 men with newly diagnosed prostate cancer and a PSA below 10 ng/ml, only seven of them had positive scans. Five of them already had painful bones that suggested to their doctors before the scan that some spread had occurred (Lee and Oesterling, 1997, p. 389). In another series of 290 men with PSAs below 10 ng/ml undergoing radionuclide scans, none had bony spread (Gleave *et al.*, 1996, p. 708). In yet another study, none of 861 newly diagnosed men with PSAs below 20 ng/ml had any bony hot spots (Levran *et al.*, 1995, p. 778).

Because of these studies, most prostate cancer specialists order bone scans only when the initial PSA level on diagnosis is above 20 ng/ml, or when there is another reason, such as persistent pain in a particular spot, to suspect bone involvement. If a bone scan does reveal spread of the cancer then it rules out the option of radical prostatectomy, which is the surgery needed to remove the whole prostate gland, with the aim of curing the disease. Who should be offered radical prostatectomy and what it entails is described in the next chapter.

10

The Decision to Treat

Having done all the tests, which include rectal examination, a PSA measurement and an ultrasound-guided biopsy, what does the prostate team do with the results? That is the subject of this short chapter. To select the correct treatment for each newly diagnosed prostate cancer case, the specialists use what is called a 'decision tree' based on the PSA and TRUS findings.

The 'tree' starts with the finding of a raised PSA – levels above 4 ng/ml need to be further investigated, preferably first with a TRUS biopsy. This gives one of three results:

- The first is a negative result for cancer, and perhaps a low-grade prostate infection (prostatitis – see page 36). Such cases only need watching over many months to make sure that the PSA is not steadily rising. In prostatitis that responds to antibiotics, the PSA level will return to normal.
- The second is also negative for prostate cancer, but shows a 'high-grade' prostatitis. If this does not resolve on antibiotic treatment, TRUS biopsies will be repeated. They may eventually be shown to be positive for cancer, or to remain negative. Rising PSA levels tend to indicate cancer.
- The third result is a positive finding of cancer. In this case, the PSA level will be assessed along with the Gleason score from the microscope appearance from the biopsy.

It is the third result that concerns us. Men who come under the third category are split into two further groups. In one, with a PSA below 10 ng/ml and a Gleason score of 6 or below, there is very little risk of extension of the cancer beyond the prostate. These men must discuss with their doctors their treatment options, which, frankly, are either to do nothing, or to have a radical prostatectomy or undergo radiation therapy.

In the other group, with a PSA above 10 ng/ml and a Gleason score of 7 and above, there is a high risk of extension of the cancer beyond the prostate. These individuals need to have a radionuclide bone scan: they may also have a CT or MRI scan, although they are less necessary or useful in most cases. If they are found to have cancer extended beyond the prostate boundaries, then they too must discuss their treatment options with their doctors. Their choice is usually anti-hormone therapy.

All these treatments are described in the following chapters.

11

Treating Cancer Confined to the Prostate Gland – Surgery

Once the staging process described in the previous chapters has proved that the cancer is still confined to the prostate, there is a need to take action. The aim of treatment in men in this early stage of prostate cancer is cure, if possible, providing that the treatment offers them a reasonable quality of life for an acceptable number of years. It may sound shocking to you, but probably the best definition of the aims of treatment of prostate cancer was given at an International Consensus Workshop on Screening and Global Strategy for Prostate Cancer held in Belgium in 1995. It asked delegates to aim at 'affording the patient the best chance of dying of something else'.

There is considerable truth in this statement. Most men discovered to have prostate cancers confined to the gland will have hardly any problems, or even no problems, from their cancers for several years. It is not sensible to subject the older men among them, perhaps with other illnesses and a life expectancy of less than ten years, to rigorous treatments that will be uncomfortable, to say the least.

So the treatment options for early prostate cancer that has not yet spread must include doing nothing but 'watching and waiting'. If you are offered that option, do consider it seriously: it could be the best management for you, and it is not a matter of your specialists opting out of your care. Naturally, you will be asked back regularly for PSA tests, rectal examinations and, if necessary, repeat biopsies, to make sure that the tumour is not growing and threatening to spread. Once there are signs that it may start to cause symptoms and worsen your quality of life, treatment can then be started.

Today the treatment options for localized cancers like this are growing year by year. Writing in 2001, they include:

- trans-urethral resection;
- radical prostatectomy;
- external beam radiation;
- brachytherapy;
- cryotherapy;

- androgen deprivation;
- laser therapy.

Some of these treatments aim to eradicate all of the cancer tissue, others, such as androgen deprivation, do not. All of them, however, have the aim of hitting the tumour so hard that it will not threaten the man's life for such a long time that he can expect to have died naturally from other causes before that happens. Kirby, Christmas and Brawer, in their book *Prostate Cancer*, published in 2001, make the interesting point that when all these treatments have been compared for men with early prostate cancers (it is difficult to compare them in a completely unbiased way), they have similar success rates. So the choice of the treatment depends at least as much on the quality of life the man enjoys after the treatment has started as on the chances of saving his life.

Trans-urethral resection: To be frank, trans-urethral resection of the prostate is an operation designed for BPH, not cancer. It is only used in older men who have bladder outflow symptoms because they have both BPH and a small prostate cancer close to the urethra, i.e. in the transition zone, which is the usual site of BPH (see Chapter 1). It is not an option for prostate cancers in the peripheral zone (the most common site for cancer) or in men with no bladder outflow problems.

Radical prostatectomy: This operation has been much more widely performed in North America than in Britain or Northern Europe, although it is gaining ground in the United Kingdom. It is confined to men in whom there is a good chance of complete cure by removing the whole prostate gland at operation. They therefore must fulfil the following criteria:

- They must have only T1 or T2 disease (see Chapter 6 for staging).
- They must be closely investigated for possible metastases and spread into the abdomen.
- They must be relatively healthy otherwise, with no signs of other serious diseases.
- They should have a life expectancy of more than ten years.

These conditions may sound harsh, but the operation is an extensive one, requiring great surgical skill, and the patient may pass through an unpleasant and fairly stormy period immediately after it. It is not one to be contemplated by someone who is older and not in the best of health. On the other hand, if it is a success, it has the huge advantage over other treatments that it gives you the security of knowing that the whole tumour has been removed and will not come back. It is then a true cure and takes much of the anxiety out of the years that follow. It is also a cure for BPH, in the many men who have both prostate diseases.

Before the operation you will have a chest X-ray, an electrocardiogram, and blood tests to ensure that the kidneys are normal and there is no anaemia. You may be asked to donate two or three units of your own blood beforehand, so that it can be transfused back into you during and after the operation. This is 'autologous' transfusion, and is being used more often in these days of fears (mostly unfounded in countries like the United Kingdom) about contaminated donor blood. Just before the operation you will start taking an antibiotic to prevent infection during surgery from bowel bacteria.

The prostate is removed either through the abdomen or via the perineum, the space between the back of the scrotum and the front of the anus. The latter is a historic route into the pelvis. The old song about Frère Jacques was about a real person, a 'cutter for the stone', who travelled Europe removing bladder stones by inserting his knife and gripping tongs into the bladder through the perineum. He must have had great success, to judge from the numbers of countries whose folklore includes him. The trend today is to use the abdominal route, rather than the perineal one.

Very great care is taken not just to remove the whole prostate, within which is the whole cancer, but also to preserve two important functions – urinary continence and the man's power of erection. This means not disturbing the nerves and blood vessels running around each side of the prostate towards the base of the penis, which are essential to erection. If the tumour is close to them, this may not be possible. It also means very careful reconstruction of the structures around the base of the bladder once the prostate is removed, so that the bladder responds normally to the message that it is becoming full, and is able to contain, without leaking, the volume of urine above it. Preserving the 'sphincter' (the muscle that closes around the top of the urethra to shut off the exit from the bladder) in this way is technically very difficult.

Radical prostatectomy has its disadvantages. It is a major operation and even in the best series of operations, published by experienced surgical teams who have done virtually nothing else for years, there are occasional unwanted complications. One is urethral stricture, in which the outflow from the bladder is partly obstructed by scarring that leaves the upper part of the urethra too narrow. It can be very uncomfortable, but it can be dealt with relatively easily. A complication that is more worrying is leakage of urine that can become serious incontinence. There are far fewer cases of incontinence after prostatectomy now that the techniques have become more refined and the anatomy around the base of the bladder is better understood.

In the past, every patient undergoing radical prostatectomy was impotent afterwards, as the nerves to the penis were routinely cut in the removal of the gland. Today, the surgeons know much more about the distribution of these nerves and how they work, and have techniques to identify them and to avoid cutting them. The result is that most men who need to retain their sexual activity can do so, and now that we have the drug sildenafil (Viagra) we can help those who have become impotent too.

How successful is radical prostatectomy? The latest series of long-term studies of men after this operation show that they survive as long as men of similar age without prostate cancer. It is difficult to beat that! These excellent results stem from the fact that the men undergoing the operations are chosen because they have tumours considered to be curable, and are therefore healthier (and often younger) than men with more extensive disease. The results are also so good because surgeons are specializing more in this type of surgery, which hones their skills and knowledge. The care immediately after surgery is also better, especially the management of postoperative pain and healing. It is so good, in fact, that the average man stays in hospital only two and a half days after the operation.

Some prostate cancer centres give their patients anti-androgen treatment for some weeks before they perform the radical prostatectomy. Anti-androgen therapy is explained in Chapters 14 and 15, as its main use is in men whose cancers have metastasized before diagnosis, but its principle is that it will shrink the cancers, because the individual cancer cells depend on androgens (testosterone and dihydrotestosterone) for their growth.

Reports on the use of anti-androgens before surgery have been uniformly good. The surgeons report at operation that, after anti-androgen treatment, the prostate is much smaller than it was at diagnosis and its margins are much clearer. This makes it easier to dissect it away from the crucial nerves and blood vessels that promote erection, and to preserve urinary continence. They also report just as good long-term survival rates as surgeons who operate earlier without a period of anti-androgen therapy. However, the experts are still divided on whether or not to give anti-androgens before surgery. The debate should be settled by two trials, one in Europe (Witjes et al., 1997, p. 65), and one in North America (Soloway et al., 1995, p. 424). They are comparing the long-term survival of men who have had radical prostatectomy with and without previous anti-androgen therapy. So far, there has been no difference between them, but it will be some years before we can compare their long-term survival.

Of course, some men who have had prostatectomies do develop recurrent cancers later, probably because some small areas of cancer outside the prostate were not recognized, or even detectable, at the time of operation. The first sign of such recurrence is a rise in PSA level, so everyone who has had a prostatectomy for cancer must return for repeated PSA tests for the rest of their lives. Around a third of men whose PSA level doubles within six months of their operation may eventually develop a recurrence. This compares with around one in six of men in whom the PSA doubles 18 months after their surgery.

Local recurrence like this may frighten you, but it must be put into perspective. In ten large-scale studies of men after radical prostatectomy for cancer, the recurrence rate over the next 15 years or so ranged from 8 per cent to a maximum of 31 per cent (Kirby, Christmas and Brawer, 2001, Table 9.11). In most of the studies, the recurrence rates were around 10 per cent. This is astonishingly good for a cancer operation of any organ, and it has to be considered in the context that even a recurrent cancer can still be treated very successfully by anti-androgen therapy. It is by no means a death sentence. We do not just have one shot at the target: radical prostatectomy is just the first of many treatments we can use.

So who should be offered it? The accepted expert view today is that it should be the first choice in younger, fitter men whose cancer is localized to the prostate, and who have reasonable expectations of living for at least another ten years. But they must be fully informed about the risks and benefits. One question they may well ask is, 'Is radical prostatectomy a better option for me than the wait and see policy mentioned at the start of this chapter?'

We do not yet know the answer. Two trials are under way, in Sweden and in the United States, in which newly diagnosed men with prostate cancer that has not yet spread beyond the gland itself are being allocated either to radical prostatectomy or to 'wait and see'. They will then be followed until their eventual deaths, from whatever cause. It sounds grisly, but it is the only way to discover which policy can save lives or improve the quality of life. We may not have the results before 2015.

12
Radiation Therapy

Radiation therapy is another option for men with localized prostate cancer. It is offered to the same men who are offered radical prostatectomy. They have cancer confirmed by biopsy that, as far as is known, is confined to the prostate. They, too, should be relatively younger men who would normally expect to have at least ten years of healthy life ahead of them.

Radiation therapy has the big advantage of offering a cure without surgery. As prostatectomy is a major operation with all the usual risks, this advantage cannot be underestimated. However, it has its disadvantages. First of all it does not help BPH, so it can leave men with bladder outflow problems that still need treatment, and perhaps TURP (see page 37). The radiation can injure the nearby bowel and bladder, so that some men who have had it need operations to repair the damage. A small number have been reported, for example, to need a colostomy (a bowel opening in the front of the abdomen) because the radiation has damaged the rectum.

Radiation treatments take a long time – they need many sessions in the radiotherapy department, which can be daunting. Unlike radical prostatectomy, radiation therapy leaves the prostate behind, so that there is a potential for future cancers to develop, and for men to remain anxious about it. Of course, there is also the objection that, like radical prostatectomy, the radiation therapy may not be needed, because the tumour will not grow fast enough or spread wide enough to cause serious illness or death.

Reading the two paragraphs above would put anyone off considering radiation treatment, but they should be put in context. Today, before you have any form of treatment, you must be fully informed about its possible disadvantages: this is as relevant to radiation therapy as it is to surgery. That is why everyone considering radiation therapy should know what can go wrong. The converse is that a lot can go right.

The main form of radiation therapy using an 'external beam', when given to the appropriate men, has excellent survival rates. Major American studies have reported more than half of their men surviving healthily for more than 15 years (Hanks, 1991, p. 231). This is similar to survival after radical prostatectomy and also to the

15-year survival rates in men of similar age without known prostate cancer. In other words, most men who have radiation therapy for their prostate cancer can look forward to living a normal and long life.

Those American figures, published in the early 1990s, relate to radiation treatments given in the 1970s. Today's techniques, in which the radiation beam is much more focused on the tumour itself and causes much less radiation damage to nearby tissues, should offer even better results and many fewer complications than those of a generation ago. Nowadays, too, many prostate cancer specialists offer, along with the radiation, surgery to remove possibly affected lymph glands in the pelvis. Such surgery is much less complex and serious than radical prostatectomy, and may 'catch' the few men with early spread that is not detectable under the usual tests.

Once you have had your radiation therapy, what then? You will be under surveillance for the rest of your life. You may be asked to have occasional needle biopsies, and you must have repeated PSA tests, to make sure that the cancer is not returning. The PSA does not fall so fast or to such low levels after radiation as after radical prostatectomy, partly because the prostate gland is still there, and some of the normal cells are still functioning (radiation 'takes out' the cancer cells selectively). However, men whose PSA levels drop below 1 ng/ml after radiation have a much lower chance of a recurrence than those whose PSA remains above 4 ng/ml.

Failure rates of around 10 per cent after conventional external beam radiation have led some centres to use new methods to deliver a higher dose of radiation more accurately and more selectively to the tumour. One of these approaches is 'conformal radiation', in which a CT scan is used to make a three-dimensional model of the prostate, and the radiation beam is 'shaped' to conform exactly to its outline. This appears to be not only more effective but also leaves fewer and less serious side effects than other radiation techniques. Other research institutes are using different types of radiation to kill the tumour cells, among them 'fast neutrons', protons and photons. Early results suggest that they all have very high response and cure rates, but they will not be widely available for some years yet.

Probably the biggest advance in radiation therapy is its use along with anti-androgen hormone therapy. The combination is thought to have two benefits. One is that any tumour cells that survive the radiation cannot multiply because they are being hit by the hormone effect (see Chapter 14 for an explanation). The other is that depriving the tumour cells of their androgen stimulus while at the same time exposing them to radiation is a double blow that may well kill them.

The results of trials of this combination of radiation followed by four months of androgen blockade have been published by the Radiation Therapy Oncology Group (RTOG) in two large studies. The first reported that in 93 per cent of the men their tumours were completely eradicated: they showed no recurrence up to at least two years later (Pilepich, 1990, p. 461). The second compared radiation only with radiation plus anti-androgen treatment in men with disease that had advanced beyond the prostate into the pelvis (Pilepich, 1995, p. 616). In these men, for whom complete cure is unlikely, by five years the disease had spread in 46 per cent of the men on combined treatment and in 71 per cent of those who had only had radiation. Twice as many men were completely free of their disease in the combined treatment group (36 per cent) than in the radiation-only group (15 per cent) after five years. These may seem low percentages, but do remember that the men concerned already had advanced disease before they had their treatment.

The best news of all comes from the European Organization for Research and Treatment of Cancer (EORTC). It compared radiation treatment alone with radiation plus anti-androgen treatment. Over the following three years there was complete local prostate disease control in 95 per cent of the men given the combined treatment and 75 per cent of those given radiation alone. Eighty-five per cent of the men on the combined treatment were metastases-free, compared with 48 per cent of the radiation-only group. Figures like these have led to a consensus that all men undergoing radiation treatment for prostate cancer should also have anti-androgen treatment for at least four months afterwards.

To summarize on treatments for early cancer that has not spread outside the gland into the pelvis or distantly:

- The final decision on whether to offer surgery or radiation, plus anti-androgen treatment, depends not just on the cancer specialist, but on you, the patient, and your family. You cannot make the decision without full information about your particular cancer and the risks and benefits of treatment. They differ from person to person, and you can only make an informed decision about whether to go ahead with a particular treatment if you know all the facts. You may only need to wait and see. You may need surgery or radiation therapy. You probably also need anti-androgen therapy. The decision ultimately depends on the discussion you have with your prostate cancer specialist.

13

Other Treatments for Localized Prostate Cancer

The vast majority of men with localized prostate cancer who need active treatment, rather than being left to 'wait and see', are treated either with radical prostatectomy or radiation therapy plus anti-androgens. With this treatment, these men do well. However, natural anxieties about the unwanted effects of these treatments have led to the development of alternative treatments with potentially fewer and less severe side effects, and with, it is hoped, the same – or an even better – success rate.

Brachytherapy

Probably the most used of these other treatments is brachytherapy. Brachytherapy has a long history, dating from 1909, when Parisian doctors Pasteau and Degrais reported their use of radium capsules, which they planted into the urethra of men with prostate cancer (Pasteau and Degrais, 1914, p. 396). The capsules were soon replaced by radium needles inserted into the cancers themselves, so that the source of the radiation was inside the tumour, rather than beside it. The technique of inserting sources of radioactivity into the prostate became known as brachytherapy, from the ancient Greek word *brachy*, meaning short – that is, the source was a short distance from the tumour.

Throughout the twentieth century radium was replaced by radioactive iodine. (For the technically minded, the isotope used is I^{125}, the radiation from which has a very short field of activity. Needles containing the correct dose of I^{125} could be used to plant 'seeds' of radioactive material at intervals of under 1 cm, and this would cover the whole prostate.) The aim was to give a higher dose of radiation to the tumour, but a much lower dose to the bladder and rectum nearby. The whole radiation dose is given with one insertion, so avoiding the repeated visits needed for external beam radiation, and saving the time of hospital staff and patients.

This process sounds ideal, but it had its problems. It was very difficult to 'map' the prostate adequately and to get the distribution of the needles or seeds correct. Some parts of the prostate were overdosed and others underdosed, and long-term follow-up revealed unacceptably high failure rates. When external beam radiation became much more accurate, brachytherapy fell from favour.

However, it is now being revived. Its main enthusiasts are in the team in the Northwest Prostate Institute in Seattle, in the United States, led by Drs Haakon Ragde and Michael Brawer. They use ultrasound systems to guide the needles carrying the 'seeds' of radioactive material into exactly the correct sites. Some patients, mainly those with low-grade cancers, are given I^{125}. Others with cancers that appear more actively multiplying when examined under the microscope are given palladium[103], a radio-isotope that decays faster than I^{125}. It can be given in a much higher dose because the time of radiation is so much shorter, with the result of a greater 'tumour-kill' in men whose cancers are highly active and multiplying fast.

The Northwest team use this form of brachytherapy for men in stage T1 or T2 disease thought to be localized to the prostate. Not all men are suitable for it. The needles are inserted through the skin of the perineum. If the prostate is very large, the pelvic bones can make it difficult for the surgeon to place the needles in the ideal pattern. Such men may need anti-androgen treatment first, to shrink their prostates before they can be given their brachytherapy. Most men who have had a previous TURP for BPH are unsuitable for brachytherapy because there is not enough prostate tissue left into which the seeds can be planted correctly. In men at high risk of spread of their cancer, who have large tumours, a high Gleason score, and high PSA levels, the Northwest team first use external beam radiation and follow it up with brachytherapy two weeks later. The implants are inserted under general or spinal anaesthesia, so that the procedure is painless and even relatively comfortable.

Most men can go home within three hours of their brachytherapy. They may need standard everyday painkillers for a few hours afterwards, but it is remarkably free of after-effects, except for, perhaps, some blood in the urine. They may need drugs to ease the flow of urine from the bladder for about a month.

In the past, people with inserted radium seeds were excluded from close company for a considerable time, because they were sources of radiation that might be dangerous to others. With modern brachytherapy, the radiation is almost completely confined to the prostate gland, so that such precautions are not needed. However, to be absolutely safe, men with seeds inserted should avoid close contact with pregnant women or with young children for two months. They may start having sex again after two weeks, providing they use a condom on the first few occasions to collect any seeds that may have migrated into the semen. Follow-up is the same as for radical prostatectomy and external beam radiation: after one month, then three-monthly, then annually after 19 months. PSAs are measured regularly and a prostate biopsy taken at 18 months.

How do the results of brachytherapy compare with those of radical prostatectomy and external beam radiation? Dr Ragde and his colleagues reported their results of 147 men given brachytherapy and followed for ten years (Ragde et al., 1998, p. 989). Given that they were elderly men to begin with (they ranged from 53 to 92 years old, most being around 70 when they were treated), their results are remarkable. Sixty-seven are still alive and well with no evidence of prostate disease. Fifty-three have died, but only three of them actually died from their prostate cancers. The rest died from the usual problems associated with old age and quite unrelated to their prostate disease. This means that there were three failures (deaths due to the disease) in 147 men, defined medically as 98 per cent disease-specific survival.

This is a huge success. Of course, some of the survivors still have their prostate cancers, but few of them appear to be life-threatening or to be advancing rapidly. Most of them, too, will reach old age without having to face death from their cancers. These results are similar to those produced by radical prostatectomy and external beam radiation. They are yet another reason for men with prostate cancer to be optimistic about the future.

Cryotherapy

Prostate cancers can be frozen, as well as irradiated. Cryotherapy, or cryoablation, the use of freezing probes to destroy prostate cancer, has a history stretching back to 1964 (Gonder, 1964, p. 610). The system uses hollow tubes inserted into the appropriate parts of the prostate under ultrasound guidance, just as with brachytherapy. Liquid nitrogen is then passed along the inside of the tubes, to create an 'ice ball' at the end. Early use of cryotherapy led to promising results, but it was difficult to stop the freeze extending to the rectum and bladder, where it caused considerable and permanent damage in a few patients. Ways of fine-tuning the freezing technique are under study, but it needs far more research before it can be considered a routine treatment.

Hyperthermia

If freezing is not satisfactory, is hyperthermia (heating up the prostate) a better alternative? There are good reasons, which we need not go into here, for thinking that cancer cells are more susceptible to dying from heat than normal cells, so applying heat to the prostate may kill cancer cells while allowing the normal tissue to survive. The current technique makes use of a probe inserted into the rectum just behind the prostate, the end of which emits microwaves that will heat up the surrounding tissues to around 43 degrees Celsius for around an hour. At least six treatments are given.

It is difficult to be certain how effective hyperthermia is, because all the studies reported so far have combined it with anti-androgen treatment or with radiotherapy, so it is impossible to be sure how much each treatment contributed to the success. In one study of 44 men given hyperthermia with either anti-androgens or radiotherapy, 24 of them had disease that had spread enough to cause severe urinary symptoms (Servadio and Leib, 1991, p. 342). The hyperthermia did not cause any serious side effects and led to a big improvement in their symptoms. Only 2 of the 27 men showed any worsening of the disease four years later, and 9 of the 11 men who had follow-up biopsies were free of the disease. In another study of men who had radical prostatectomies between six and nine days after microwave heating had been applied to their prostate glands, the technique missed tumours in certain areas of the peripheral zone, which is the part of the prostate that 'grows' most cancers. So although hyperthermia has promise, it is by no means a proven reliable form of treatment. We need much larger trials and longer follow-up after treatment.

Lasers

Laser treatment is a form of hyperthermia, in that the intense light from a laser is converted into heat when it hits the target tissue. A tube is passed into the urethra to the level of the prostate. It delivers, from its 'head', laser light at right angles to its length under guidance from a fibre-optic tube. The surgeons can see exactly where they are applying the light. The result is 'coagulation' (in effect, a burn) of tissue to a depth of 3 to 4 mm. The area removed gradually shrinks into a harmless scar. The technique has mainly been used several weeks after men have had TURP for localized cancer, to 'burn' away any suspected residual prostate cancer tissue. A 1984 study reported only 7 treatment failures among 63 men two years after their laser surgery (Sander and Beisland, 1984, p. 280). Nine years later another group reported 22 of 26 men as disease-free after TURP followed by laser therapy. However, this was a relatively short follow-up, and none of the men, who all had the initial diagnosis of cancer localized to the prostate, showed the fall in PSA values to near-zero that is needed for reassurance of cure.

New laser techniques are being developed that will surely be used eventually in routine treatment of prostate cancer, but the evidence that lasers are preferable to the tried and trusted treatments for prostate cancer is still sparse. We may have to wait years before we have enough data on it to make a reasoned decision on whether or not it should be used.

Of all the alternative methods of treating prostate cancer, the one with most promise is probably brachytherapy. I look forward to writing more about it in future editions of this book.

14

Cancer Beyond the Prostate –'Locally Advanced'

As mentioned earlier in this book, prostate cancer spreads in two ways. First, it spreads through its surrounding 'capsule' (its outer 'skin'). This is defined as locally advanced prostate cancer, and this chapter deals with its treatment. Second, there is distant spread to other organs, usually bones, called 'metastatic' prostate cancer. Its treatment is described in the next chapter.

Cancers that have spread through the prostate capsule are no longer curable by even radical prostatectomy, so it is not an option. There have been a few studies of the use of surgery in men who first have three months of anti-androgen treatment, in an effort to 'down-stage' their cancers from 'locally advanced' to 'prostate only'. There are two objections to this. The first is that there is little evidence that anti-androgens will completely remove all cancer tissue outside the prostate. The second is that subjecting such men to radical surgery does not improve their long-term survival any more than does a medicine-only approach.

Using external beam radiation on its own in such men is also disappointing. Most men in trials of this technique alone for locally advanced cancer showed evidence of residual cancer afterwards. Their cancers also tended to become metastatic, so they had a poorer life expectancy than men offered other treatments. Their PSA levels, too, did not drop steeply enough to give doctors confidence that it is a complete treatment.

These findings led specialists towards devising other treatments for locally advanced cancers. The first was to add anti-androgen treatments to radiotherapy. This more than doubles the number of men who remain free of progressive cancer after five years (Pilepich, 1995, p. 616). Adding anti-androgen treatment to radiotherapy reduced the proportion of men whose cancers progressed in the next five years from 71 per cent on radiotherapy alone to 46 per cent.

The second choice is to do without the radiation, and use anti-androgen therapy alone. The decision to drop radiation from treatment in locally advanced prostate cancer comes from studies in which anti-androgen alone has had good results, without the complications that can arise from radiation (see Chapter 12).

Anti-androgen therapy

The first anti-androgen was the female sex hormone, oestrogen. Giving oestrogen to a man with prostate cancer shuts down the production of testosterone, the main male sex hormone, by the testes. As most prostate cancer cells depend on testosterone to grow and multiply, this arrests the progress of the cancer, and leaves the cells open to 'apoptosis', the process in which cells 'commit suicide'. Oestrogen treatment did ease the symptoms of prostate cancer, but at the expense of feminizing the man, so that he grew feminine breasts, lost all sexual desire, and became impotent. It was a high price to pay for a treatment that in the end was not a cure.

Castration, by removing the testes at operation, was introduced in the 1940s. It had far fewer side effects. The prostate gland no longer has the stimulus of testosterone, and without the extra oestrogen the man does not turn into a pseudo-female. Castration is highly successful: it checks the growth of cancer, reducing the volume of the growth by more than 60 per cent, and often by 80 per cent in almost every case. For locally advanced cancers inside the pelvis, this means there is much less pressure on the bladder, urethra and rectum. Men who had the operation felt much better within hours of the operation. Their bladder outflow problems, their pelvic and abdominal tenderness, difficulties with bowel movements, and feelings of general ill health, are almost instantaneously relieved. The operation itself is a relatively minor one, usually performed under a local or spinal anaesthetic, and causes much less discomfort than radiation. A few men are bruised afterwards, and even fewer have minor infections at the site of the operation (these can be readily dealt with).

Naturally, castration has its major drawbacks, not least the understandable reluctance that any man would feel at losing his testes. After castration, most men lose their sexual feelings and become impotent: in men with a good sex life its loss can seem worse than death itself. And castration is irreversible.

Happily there are now excellent medical, reversible, alternatives to castration that do exactly the same thing – remove the ability of the testes to produce testosterone. These are drugs that fall into two classes: pure anti-androgens, and 'LHRH agonists'. They need a chapter of their own to describe how they act in the body (see Chapter 15). For the purposes of this chapter, bearing in mind that it is about locally advanced prostate cancer without distant metastases, these drugs can be used instead of castration, and have the benefit of being able to be used in intermittent 'bursts' of treatment. The most commonly used anti-androgen drugs for locally advanced cancers are bicalutamide (Casodex), flutamide (Drogenil), leuprorelin acetate (Prostap), goserelin (Zoladex), and buserelin (Suprefact).

Why should they be used intermittently? Some researchers believe that giving anti-androgens constantly to men with locally advanced cancer may increase the risk that the cancer cells may become able to multiply in the absence of androgens. In medical terms they become 'androgen-independent', and therefore much more difficult to control. Androgen-independent cancers no longer respond to anti-androgen treatment, and need different types of chemotherapy. It would be far better to avoid this development. One way to do this, according to the new view, is to deprive the cancer of androgen enough to drive the PSA level below 4 ng/ml, and to keep it there for 32 weeks. The man should then be considered for stopping his anti-androgen treatment at the thirty-sixth week.

Over the next 8 to 14 weeks his testes will start to work again, and his testosterone level, and his PSA level, will gradually climb until they are back to their pre-treatment figures. The general rule is that if the man's PSA level is under 20 ng/ml at first diagnosis, then the next course of anti-androgen drugs is started when the PSA has returned to that first measurement. If the initial PSA was above 20 ng/ml (and it can be in the thousands), then the next course of anti-androgens is started when the PSA (having fallen to near zero after the first course of treatment) has returned to 20 ng/ml.

This second course of treatment continues until the PSA has fallen again to near zero, and carries on for another 32 weeks before the treatment is again stopped. The next cycle of treatment is again started only after the PSA has risen as after the first cycle. Many patients go through five or more of these treatment cycles with no evidence of any advance in the tumour, and most show real shrinkage of their cancers.

These repeated courses of anti-androgen therapy interspersed with periods of no treatment have several advantages. They may prevent cancers from becoming androgen-independent and therefore resistant to treatment. Just as important, they improve the man's quality of life. Stopping the drugs causes any side effects to disappear. The men recover their sexual feelings (that are almost always lost on anti-androgens), they feel generally better, and they are protected to some extent from one common complication of deprivation of androgens: the 'brittle bone disease' called osteoporosis. It is difficult to know for sure that intermittent anti-androgen therapy is better than constant anti-androgen therapy. The only evidence so far is a small trial in which the long-term results were similar to those of continuous androgen deprivation (Goldenberg, 1994, p. 240A). Trials now under way (in 2001) in many more men with localized spread of their prostate cancers will settle the question.

Treating the complications of locally advanced prostate cancer

When prostate cancers enlarge and spread into the neighbouring tissues, they tend to cause two major complications – bladder outflow problems (see page 26) and pressure on the ureter (the tube from the kidney to the bladder).

Bladder outflow problems in any man are far more likely to be due to benign prostatic hyperplasia (BPH – see page 26) than to locally advanced cancer, and the usual treatment is TURP (see page 37). However, TURP often leads to urinary incontinence (mainly constant leakage of urine) when it is done for cancer, rather than for BPH. Most prostate specialists would therefore prefer to shrink malignant obstructions with anti-androgens instead of operating. Unhappily for the men, while they are on this treatment they need to be catheterized (with a permanent drainage tube from the bladder to the penis). One way to avoid this is to place a 'stent' (a small section of tubing) inside the urethra to keep the narrowed section open. Most people do not notice that their stent is in place, and can urinate normally, but some find it painful and uncomfortable, and it can lead to bladder infections. Stents can also move upwards into the bladder or downwards and out during urination, so they need close supervision while they are in place. After around three months, when the prostate has shrunk enough for normal urination to resume, the stent can be removed.

Stents can also be inserted into an obstructed ureter for the same reason – pressure by an expanding tumour or by nearby enlarged lymph glands on the back of the bladder. If it is impossible to do this, the next step is to bring the affected ureter out on to the abdominal wall, so as to ease the back-pressure on the kidney on that side. This is called a nephrostomy.

Very rarely (thankfully, because it is a miserable condition) prostate cancers grow locally so large that they wrap themselves around the bowel behind them, making the man extremely consti-pated and uncomfortable (he feels as if he is always needing to empty his bowel, but cannot, no matter how hard he strains). Although anti-androgen treatment may help these men a lot, some eventually need a colostomy (a bowel opening on the front of the abdomen) to give them relief.

15

Cancer Beyond the Prostate – Metastatic Disease

By the time prostate cancer has spread distantly, with metastases in bones and other organs, surgery is no longer an option. First and foremost, if the multiple tumour sites are to be hit hard, the man needs 'androgen ablation' – the removal of all influence that androgens such as testosterone exert on the tumour cells. As is the case for men with cancer that has spread only within the pelvis (see Chapter 14), the options are either castration or the use of anti-androgen drugs.

This is probably the right place to describe how the two main types of anti-androgen drugs work. The first ones to be developed were the 'LHRH agonists'. LHRH (the initials stand for Luteinizing Hormone Releasing Hormone) agonists are drugs that cause the pituitary gland to pour out LHRH into the bloodstream. Luteinizing Hormone Releasing Hormone is a confusing name for the hormone in men, because it relates to its action in women. Another, probably more appropriate, name for LHRH is gonadorelin, so that LHRH agonists are also called gonadorelin agonists.

To understand how LHRH agonists work, one must know a little about the way the pituitary gland regulates the release of sex hormones by the ovary and the testes. Luteinizing hormone (LH) is released by the pituitary gland (it hangs down from the base of the brain inside the skull) into the bloodstream. In women, LH is released mainly in mid-menstrual cycle, and it causes the ovary, in turn, to release the hormone progesterone into the bloodstream, and to 'drop' an egg into the uterus, ready for fertilization. If conception takes place, then the progesterone prepares the lining of the womb to receive the fertilized egg by initiating the first stages of the formation of the placenta, the organ through which the developing infant is nourished and by which it is anchored to the womb. In the meantime the spot on the surface of the ovary from which the egg has fallen becomes the 'corpus luteum' (yellow body). The corpus luteum produces the hormone human chorionic gonadotrophin (hCG) that then sustains the pregnancy by helping it to firmly embed into the wall of the womb.

Luteinizing hormone was therefore named in this way because it led to the formation of the corpus luteum. It was only later discovered that exactly the same pituitary hormone is used in men to cause the testes to produce testosterone. Without the message of LH from the pituitary, the testes produce no testosterone, and the man is 'medically castrated'.

Now we have to go one step back in the biochemical chain. LH is only produced by the pituitary if it is told to do so by another hormone, produced by an area of brain just above it called the hypothalamus. This hormone is called LHRH, Luteinizing Hormone Releasing Hormone, for the elementary reason that it causes the pituitary to release LH into the bloodstream, from which the testes pick up the message to produce testosterone.

So far, so good. But why give an LHRH agonist if you wish to stop the testes from producing testosterone? Logic suggests that it will make the testes produce more testosterone, not less. That is true. Give an LHRH agonist to a man and there is a fast rise in testosterone levels to around 150 per cent of normal. But within 21 days of starting continuous treatment with an LHRH agonist, testosterone levels plummet to near zero, to the levels seen after castration. This is because constant exposure to LHRH switches off the pituitary's response, and it no longer produces LH. The testes have no stimulus to produce testosterone, so they stop producing it. And they will not start producing it again until the LHRH agonist treatment is stopped.

LHRH agonists

As with locally advanced prostate cancer (see the previous chapter), the LHRH agonists used for metastatic cancer include buserelin (Suprefact), goserelin (Zoladex), leuprorelin acetate (Prostap) and triptorelin (Decapeptyl).

Buserelin is unique among them in that in long-term use it is delivered by nasal spray. For the first week it is given by three daily injections under the skin: then the man changes to the spray, giving himself six sprays a day from then on. Goserelin is given by a solid rod implant, delivered through a wide bored needle, under the skin of the front of the abdomen. It can be given as Zoladex once a month or as Zoladex LA once every 12 weeks. Leuprorelin is given as an injection of 'microspheres' through a syringe under the skin either as Prostap SR once a month or as Prostap 3 once every three months. Triptorelin is also given as a microsphere injection of Decapeptyl sr, once every four weeks. Microspheres are tiny spheres containing the drug, designed to release a steady amount of it into the surrounding tissues over the month between injections.

LHRH agonists must be given in these ways because when they are swallowed they are digested and therefore would not work.

Direct anti-androgens

The second type of anti-androgen includes cyproterone acetate (Cyprostat), bicalutamide (Casodex), and flutamide (Droganil). There is also nilutamide (Anandrone), which is not in use in Britain. These 'direct' anti-androgens do not work on LHRH. Instead they block the formation of testosterone by both the testes and of dihydrotestosterone by the adrenal glands. As mentioned in Chapter 3, the adrenal glands, which sit above the kidneys, produce a small amount of androgen.

Using both types of anti-androgen – together

Now comes the difficult bit: how can these two types of anti-androgen be used to the maximum benefit in men with metastatic prostate cancer? There is no argument among the experts on the first way in which they are used – on the day of diagnosis and for the next three weeks. However, the experts are keenly (even fiercely) divided on how they should be used after that.

The main aim of the initial treatment of metastatic prostate cancer is to remove the influence of testosterone as fast and as effectively as possible. However, just giving an LHRH agonist alone would mean exposing the man to a week or so of higher, rather than lower, blood levels of testosterone, before they began to fall. This can make the symptoms worse for a while, as the cancer cells become more active. It can lead to more intense bone pain, and make the man feel more ill. If he has a metastasis in one of his vertebrae, the consequent swelling can put pressure on the spinal cord. Such spinal cord compression can lead to weakness and paralysis, so it must be avoided at all costs. These increasing symptoms immediately after starting men on LHRH agonists is called a 'flare', and it can last up to three weeks.

The flare phenomenon is why, for those first three weeks, men with metastases at the time of diagnosis need both types of anti-androgen. Either cyproterone acetate or flutamide is given along with the LHRH agonist. They prevent the initial rise in testosterone that LHRH agonist would cause, so avoiding the flare. Then, as the long-term effect of the LHRH agonist 'kicks in', the direct anti-androgen can be stopped.

This is where the controversy starts. What should be done next? The argument revolves around whether the direct anti-androgens should be continued, along with the LHRH agonist, or whether it is better for the LHRH agonist to be given on its own. Some experts believe the two should be continued together, to make sure that even the smallest amount of androgen in the blood, including both testosterone and the androgens made in the adrenal gland, is abolished. This 'maximal androgen blockade' has been pioneered by Dr Fernand Labrie and his colleagues in Quebec. Dr Labrie is a real enthusiast for the dual treatment, and it is only fair to say that I have been present at meetings in which the debate for and against his methods has been spirited, to say the least.

His argument goes like this. Just blocking the androgen (testosterone) produced by the testes using an LHRH agonist leaves untouched the androgen (DHT, or dihydrotestosterone – see page 17) produced by the adrenal glands. Dr Labrie and his colleagues say that the adrenal androgen may still stimulate prostate cancer cells, and that this stimulation should be switched off by adding a direct anti-androgen such as flutamide to the LHRH agonist. They say that the combined drugs give a better initial response in more men, delay the time to the tumour developing androgen independence (see the last chapter), lengthen the time to the cancer starting to increase again (defined as cancer progression), and improve survival rates.

The argument against Dr Labrie's approach is that giving both types of drug together over long periods increases the patient's side effects and is a considerable extra cost. These objections may not be too important if the combination of the two types of drug does actually improve life quality and length of survival, but are very important if it does not. So it is incumbent upon supporters of Dr Labrie's management to prove that it does what is claimed for it.

Have they proved their point? It is still difficult to say, although recent studies are increasingly suggesting support for them. The Quebec team's first published study in 1985 showed such good figures on combined treatment that they were hardly believed by the other prostate cancer researchers at the time. Only one of 87 patients with metastatic cancer died within two years of the diagnosis, and only eight of the cancers had progressed (Labrie, 1985, p. 833). These figures are considerably better than comparable studies using LHRH agonists alone, and they led to many more studies being undertaken.

Some of them tended to support the Quebec team, but others found no difference in survival, or in time to recurrence of the disease, between the combined treatment and the use of LHRH agonists alone. It must be admitted that almost all of the trials showed that the two-pronged attack on the cancer led to a longer delay to signs of recurrence of the cancer, but not necessarily to a longer life. When the Prostate Cancer Trialists Collaborative Group (PCTCG) examined 22 trials involving 5,710 men, the estimated risk of death was between 6 and 22 per cent lower with maximum androgen blockade than after castration alone (PCTCG, 1995, p. 265). Although surgical castration is not the same as LHRH agonist treatment alone, it has a very similar effect.

One way to judge treatment effectiveness is to measure the men's PSA levels. When 411 men were treated either with leuprolide plus placebo or leuprolide plus flutamide, 76 per cent of the men on the two drugs, but only 52 per cent of the men on leuprolide plus placebo, reached normal PSA levels within three months (Smith, 1991, p. 384A). This is fairly strong evidence that the combination may be more effective in shutting down cancer activity.

Where do I stand in the debate? First of all this is my own opinion, not necessarily the correct one, and probably not one shared by most prostate cancer consultants. It has been formed from what I have read and from conversations with cancer specialists, and not from personal experience of treating hundreds of men with prostate cancer. A general practitioner like myself will only see a few new cases per year, so any judgement from my own experience can only be anecdotal. For what it is worth, however, if I have the misfortune to have the disease myself, and it is metastatic from the start, I would wish to have maximum androgen blockade, with (at the moment) flutamide or bicalutamide and one of the LHRH agonists. My view may change as trial results are published in the future. Many consultants still hold to the view that adding a direct anti-androgen to LHRH agonist treatment is only adding side effects, and not extra life or quality of life. I fully respect that view, and would ask men faced with the decision on management of their tumours to discuss openly with their consultant the difference between the two treatments, and their relevance to their special case. There may be good reasons for either treatment in any individual case.

In Britain the official position is that LHRH agonists are licensed for use alone for metastatic prostate cancer, and the direct anti-androgens cyproterone acetate, flutamide, and bicalutamide are licensed for use in preventing flare in the first three weeks of LHRH agonist treatment. Cyproterone acetate and flutamide are also licensed for use on their own as treatment for prostate cancer that has progressed on LHRH agonist treatment. So far, bicalutamide is licensed only for locally advanced, non-metastatic cancer, and not yet for metastatic cancer. This may change soon, as the results of current large trials of its use in metastatic cancer are reported. In any case, each prostate specialist is free to prescribe what he thinks is needed by each patient.

Side effects of anti-androgens

If you read the list of side effects on the inserts inside the packages of the various anti-androgen drugs, you will probably be shocked at their number and severity. However, do understand that this is an extensive list covering every side effect that has been reported, and that most of them are rare. Side effects that are not rare, however, are the ones that are caused by the drugs' main actions, such as testosterone suppression.

LHRH agonists, because they have such strong effects on hormone levels, produce symptoms very similar to menopausal problems in women. Common ones are hot flushes, drenching sweats, loss of sexual desire, and impotence. Much less common are rashes, itch and, extremely rarely, asthma and severe allergic reactions. Some men have a red, swollen irritating reaction around the injection site. Other very occasional reactions include headache, migraine, hair loss, dizziness, muscle and joint pains, swelling of the ankles, indigestion, weight changes (up and down), difficulties in sleeping, and swings in mood.

Taking direct anti-androgens along with LHRH agonists can make all these symptoms worse. They may also add a risk of liver problems, including jaundice, abnormal heart rhythms, a tendency towards diabetes, pain in the pelvis, anaemia, and bleeding disorders. Nilutamide, for example, can make it more difficult for you to adapt your vision quickly when going between light and dark environments, and can lower your tolerance to alcohol.

81

Cyproterone acetate differs from other direct anti-androgens in that it is a 'progestogen'. When given over many months the testes overcome the drug's ability to suppress testosterone formation, so that testosterone levels tend to rise again. As cyproterone's side effects include an increased risk of thrombosis (blood clots in veins) and a tendency to induce diabetes, as well as to cause liver problems, it is used only for short periods unless it is a last resort when all else has failed.

Other ways to maximal androgen suppression

There are times when LHRH agonists and direct anti-androgens have failed or are no longer appropriate, or need supporting by other drugs that may also block androgens. One is aminoglutethamide (Orimeten). It not only blocks the formation of androgen, but also the production of other steroid hormones such as cortisone (cortisol) and of aldosterone, a hormone that helps to control salt levels in the body, and therefore blood pressure. So men given aminoglutetha-mide for their prostate cancer must also be given a cortisone-like drug such as prednisolone to keep various vital processes, including the blood pressure, normal. Aminoglutethamide is not an easy drug to take, particularly in the first two weeks, when it often makes you sleepy, raises your temperature, and gives you a rash. These effects usually settle on their own, but other more serious side effects can arise with longer treatment. They mean that men on lasting aminoglutethamide treatment must have frequent checks on their blood pressure, and blood tests to check on the possible development of anaemia, loss of white blood cells, thyroid function, and plasma 'electrolytes'. This last is a measure of aldosterone blockade and is intimately linked to blood pressure and kidney function. Not surprisingly, aminoglutethamide is reserved very much as a second- or third-line treatment for prostate cancer.

A drug that is used widely to 'shrink' prostate tissue in benign prostatic hyperplasia (BPH), finasteride (Proscar), may find a use in men with prostate cancer too, provided it is always given with, rather than instead of, an anti-androgen. Many men have both BPH and prostate cancer, and there is some evidence from animal studies that it may have anti-tumour activity as well as the ability to reduce benign overgrowth of prostate tissue. It blocks the final stage from testosterone to dihydrotestosterone, in the process raising the levels of testosterone within the gland. In one trial in men who had residual prostate cancer after radical prostatectomy, giving finasteride delayed the subsequent rise in PSA by about 18 months (Andriole, 1994, p. 450A). When given with flutamide it was as effective in keeping rises in PSA at bay as goserelin plus flutamide (Kirby, 1999, p. 105). At present, however, finasteride is not recommended officially for prostate cancer: whether that will change soon depends, as is usual with new uses of drugs, on the results of ongoing trials.

Summarizing management of metastatic prostate cancer – the picture in 2001

The first-line treatment for prostate cancer that has spread to distant sites is to remove androgens either by castration or by using LHRH agonists. The trend is away from surgical castration towards medical 'castration' with LHRH agonists, with the proviso that in the first three weeks a direct anti-androgen is used to prevent flare. Many specialists are turning towards maximal androgen removal using both an LHRH agonist and a direct anti-androgen long term, particularly in fitter and younger men in whom it could be expected that they could live long enough eventually to die from, rather than with, their cancer (Kirby, 1994, p. 31). In older men, there may be good reason to use an LHRH agonist on its own, to minimize the side effects that are more common on the two-drug system.

There is huge optimism that the near future will bring drugs that can be taken by mouth that will not only avoid the need for surgery or injections, but also allow men taking them to have a normal sex life. It is also important to recognize that for men who already have metastatic cancer there is not the choice of 'wait and see' that is described in Chapter 10. That policy is confined to cancers that have not spread beyond the limits of the prostate. Once the cancer has spread, LHRH agonists with or without a direct anti-androgen are essential to deal with the symptoms and to prevent further spread of the disease.

16

Dealing with Androgen Independence

Unfortunately there comes a time when even some expertly treated prostate cancers become androgen-independent. Despite continuing complete androgen blockade, the cancer begins to spread again, and further anti-androgen and LHRH treatment no longer helps. The first sign of this development is a rise in PSA despite continuing low testosterone levels. Sometimes, paradoxically, this rise is arrested and even reversed by stopping the anti-androgen therapy. Experts in the field believe that this is because some of the cells have mutated, so that they are now stimulated, rather than stunned, by the anti-androgen. So the first action in someone taking, for example, flutamide plus an LHRH agonist, and whose PSA is rising, is to stop the flutamide. That may be all that is needed to slow or stop the cancer progressing.

If that action fails, then the next step is to use one of two different approaches. One is to use drugs that increase oestrogen levels in the blood. There is some evidence that oestrogen will directly harm prostate cancer cells. One oestrogen used in this way is the straightforward oestrogen diethylstilboestrol (DES). It may keep the cancer at bay for many months, but only at the price of side effects such as the development of feminine breasts. It is also linked to deep vein thrombosis and heart problems, but these can be prevented by taking just one 75 mg aspirin a day.

A more complex oestrogen that is used more often in metastatic prostate cancer is estramustine (Estracyt). This combines in one capsule oestrogen and mustine, an anti-cancer agent. Estramustine seems to concentrate in the prostate gland where it selectively destroys cancer cells, and trials have reported that around 60 per cent of men given it after relapses on anti-androgen treatment respond well to it in terms of feeling better. In around half of them there is also good objective evidence that the tumour has responded. Unfortunately, estramustine can also affect the bone marrow, so that it can cause anaemia and damage the white cells. It also may cause nausea that does not easily respond to anti-nausea drugs. If any of these side effects occur, it has to be stopped.

Studies of other 'cytotoxic' (anti-cancer) drugs in prostate cancer that has become resistant to anti-androgens have been disappointing so far. The National Prostate Cancer Project (NPCP) in the United States has published a series of trials of different combinations of cytotoxic drugs, among them cyclophosphamide, 5-fluorouracil, streptozotin, hydroxyurea, vincristine, and cisplatin along with estramustine. The response to them has been mixed, sometimes only a little better than the response to placebo.

Growth factor inhibitors

One of the most exciting stories in medicine in the last few years has been the development of our knowledge of growth factors and their inhibitors or blockers. Growth factors are the natural substances produced by our bodies to stimulate our cells to grow normally. When cancers occur, growth factors may continue to stimulate the cells, leading to spread both locally and distantly in metastases. Once we knew about growth factors and how they affect cells, it became imperative to develop drugs that would block their actions. They fall into the category of growth factor inhibitors.

Suramin is one of these drugs. Trials of suramin in androgen-independent prostate cancer started as long ago as 1988. The first trial had excellent results, considering that the men had all eventually failed to respond to anti-androgen and LHRH agonist treatment (Myers, 1992, p. 881). Of the 38 men starting on the trial, 17 of the cancers had spread to soft tissues and 18 to bone. In one-third of the men with soft tissue spread and half of those with bone involvement, their metastases shrank. Seventy per cent of the men had much less bone pain and more than half of them showed at least a halving of their PSA. Suramin helped most those with lower (less than 100 ng/ml), rather than higher, initial PSA levels. The authors of the report concluded that there was a limit to the cancer spread beyond which suramin was of less value.

However, suramin has not gained general acceptance. It causes skin and nerve problems, and abnormal feelings in the limbs (medically, these are 'paraesthesiae') and increased susceptibility to infection, among other severe side effects. We will need to wait for growth factor blockers that are more specific to prostate cancer cells. They are surely on the way. Suramin is only a precursor drug to pave the way for others that are less dangerous.

Another drug that shows promise – because it may be the start of a new series of drugs rather than for its own merits – is paclitaxol

(Taxol), which is already used in advanced ovarian and breast cancer. It is limited by a serious adverse effect on the bone marrow, which includes the shutting down of white cell production and a much increased susceptibility to infection. Yet it did lower PSA levels in men with advanced metastatic androgen-independent prostate cancer (Roth, 1993, p. 2457). Other, less toxic, drugs in the paclitaxol mould are sure to follow it.

Palliation

There comes a time in some prostate cancer patients' lives when the aim is not necessarily to keep the cancer at bay, but to ease the symptoms that it causes. This is defined as palliation, and the symptom that most needs it is bone pain. Pain in the bone from cancer deposits may well not respond to the usual painkillers, whether they are based on aspirin, paracetamol or morphine.

However, it may respond to 'bisphosphonates'. These are drugs designed originally for women with osteoporosis, whose bones are losing calcium. Bisphosphonates are a group of drugs that direct calcium into bones and prevent calcium loss from them. They have been used successfully in bony metastases from breast cancer. One bisphosphonate, clodronate (Bonefos, or Loron), eased bone pain in 16 of 17 men given it by injection for severe bone pain caused by androgen-independent prostate cancer (Adami, 1985, p. 246). Newer bisphosphonates that are given by mouth may be just as effective.

When the bone pain is localized to one spot, radiotherapy can help a lot, given as a single dose or over several weeks. More extensive bone pain may be treated with 'wide-field' radiotherapy, in which half the body is irradiated in one dose, then the other half later. Unfortunately, wide-field radiotherapy is extremely debilitating, with more than a third of men receiving it feeling sick and having diarrhoea. It is reserved for men whose bone pain is very severe and who may wish to take the risk. It does relieve the pain completely in around 30 per cent of the men treated, and another 50 per cent report at least a partial response.

One form of radiation treatment has been useful for bone pain. It is strontium-89 (Metastron). This radioactive substance is taken up preferentially at sites where metastases are particularly active, and therefore causing most pain. It then shuts down the bone activity. A survey of several studies has reported relief of bone pain in 78 per cent of men given strontium-89 (Crawford, 1994, p. 481). Others have shown similar results. A British study in 284 men also concluded that men given strontium-89 were less likely to develop new sites of pain than others given external beam radiotherapy (Porter, 1993, p. 38).

Strontium-89 produces milder side effects than other forms of radiotherapy and cytotoxic drugs: it is given as a single dose, and its effects usually last three months or more. After that time, more doses can be given if the need arises.

If the worst happens, and all treatment eventually fails, then care must be put into the hands of a team of carers experienced in palliative care, which should include the patient's relatives, and his general practitioner. The aim of all treatment is to try to prevent the patient reaching this final stage, but it is only common sense to plan ahead. Most men naturally wish to stay at home for as long as possible, but there are times when a move to a nursing home is the sensible thing to do. It is best to organize a move like this in advance, so that the transfer is not done in a rush into a place that may not be to your liking. If this is the case for you, please heed your doctor's and nurse's advice. It may not seem like it, but this is usually the best for you: the main aim at this stage is to keep you comfortable, and the most likely way for this to happen is under the care of experienced professionals.

17

Coping with Sex

This subject has been left to last, not because it is the least important, but because sexual activity can be a problem at any stage of prostate cancer and its treatment. It is one thing to be treated successfully for prostate cancer, but quite another to have treatment that preserves the enjoyment and mechanics of a normal sex life. Men today are open about the need to preserve the quality of their sex lives and, it follows, of their partners' sex lives too.

It has to be accepted that treatments for prostate cancer do interfere with your sex life. The old operation to remove the prostate in men with early cancers divided the nerve and blood vessels to the penis, so that sexual feelings and erection were both permanently lost. The newer operations, which go to great lengths to spare both nerves and blood supply, have greatly improved the chances that after healing both sexual feeling and potency will be normal. Nevertheless, only about half of men undergoing modern radical prostatectomy return to their full sex lives afterwards.

TURP is more successful in maintaining both sexual feelings and potency, but even with this operation, in which the material removed is not near the nerves and blood supply to the penis, around 16 per cent of men have problems with starting and/or maintaining an erection afterwards. Why this happens is not clear. All forms of radiation therapy, including brachytherapy, can lead to impotence, mainly because the arteries within the prostate, which lead to the penis, are affected by the radiation. Studies suggest that around 60 per cent of men remain potent with normal sex lives after external beam radiation therapy.

Brachytherapy seems to be better at preserving potency: of 56 men in one brachytherapy study, 85 per cent of them were still potent after three years (Wallner, 1996, p. 449). On the other hand, cryotherapy has a bad record: 88 per cent of 74 men undergoing cryotherapy who had a normal sex life before treatment were impotent afterwards (Kirby, Christmas and Brawer, 2001, p. 204).

Castration (which is used less and less these days as a treatment for prostate cancer) reduces sexual desire in most men, and with it comes impotence, but not in all men. Presumably their potency depends on the androgens produced by the adrenal glands mentioned on page 16. Medical 'castration' induced by maximal androgen blockade (i.e. use of an LHRH agonist plus a direct anti-androgen) causes a complete loss of interest in sex and impotence because it removes even the small amount of androgen produced by the adrenal glands. In one Italian study (DiSilverio, 1990, p. 54), the use of goserelin and cyproterone acetate together led to 86 per cent of the men becoming impotent and losing interest in sex.

Most men, obviously, would like to retain their normal sex lives, even at the risk of a slightly higher risk of dying from their disease. This is one reason put forward for giving bicalutamide to some men with advanced cancers who wish to keep on enjoying sex. Bicalutamide is the drug, so far, that is most successful in maintaining potency in men with advanced prostate cancer. However, it is not as good as other drugs in treating metastases in bone. This is a trade-off that is difficult to measure, and should be a matter for serious discussion between patient and specialist.

Impotence can be treated without the need to put yourself at greater risk of cancer spreading. Today, you can learn to inject materials such as the drug alprostadil into the penis (using Caverject or Viridal) or into the urethra (MUSE – Medicated Urethral System for Erection) to produce an erection. You can use a vacuum device, or take sildenafil (Viagra) pills. Eighty per cent of 15 men with problems with erection after a radical prostatectomy found success with sildenafil.

Some men remain potent and have orgasms after prostate surgery, but no longer ejaculate. This is commonest after TURP, when the ejaculate goes into the bladder, rather than out through the urethra. Anyone having prostate surgery, whether it is for BPH or cancer, should be warned beforehand that this may happen. Many men who find that this is happening avoid sex: if they are warned beforehand they and their partners can usually cope. Attempts to correct the backward flow of sperm after surgery have met with little success: with guidance and advice, most men accept it as an inconvenience, rather than a disaster. The sperm is expelled with the next urination.

In the very small number of men with prostate cancer who still wish to father children, sperm can still be obtained by applying an electrical current to the nerves and blood vessels around the remaining prostate gland tissue. Whether this is desirable, considering the doubts about the future health of the father of any child born after sperm has been obtained in this way, is an ethical, not a medical, matter.

18
Hopes for the Future

Looking forward, there are signs that there will be better treatments for prostate cancer, and that their success rates will improve even more in the next few years than they have over the last 40. In health matters, the United States is often the trend setter. Since American doctors started to use PSA as a detection tool in the 1980s, far more prostate cancers than ever before have been detected in their curable early stages. Because of this, and because treatments are more effective, the numbers of deaths from prostate cancers have actually declined in the United States – an astonishing fact, considering that there are so many more older men than there used to be.

PSA tests have helped enormously to pick up the early cases before they reach stages for which cure is impossible. There may be new tests that will detect the cancers that are most likely to metastasize early, and that need more urgent treatment. One of them may be measurement of blood levels of 'E-cadherin'. Another may be the identification of genes that increase the chances of prostate cancer in families in which there have been several cases. Already two such genes are known.

There are signs, too, that radiotherapy techniques will improve to pick out only prostate cancer cells, leaving normal tissues undisturbed, and avoiding incontinence afterwards.

A whole new class of drugs, the LHRH antagonists, will soon be on the prescription lists. They will do the same as the LHRH agonists, but without the initial flare. One of them, abarelix, is going through its final trials. The early trials were very encouraging.

Another idea is 'chemoprevention', in which drugs given to men at potential risk of prostate cancer may prevent it from developing. Two candidates for this are similar to vitamins A and D. Another is the finasteride mentioned previously (see page 82) that is already widely used to reduce prostate size in BPH. Further ahead are possibilities for gene therapy, and the use of genes to enhance the body's own immune defences against cells that are beginning to turn into cancers.

Another possible way forward is to prepare 'vaccines' from chemical products of the man's own cancer cells and induce an immune response against them.

I mention all these approaches (and there are many more) to show that research into prostate cancer is expanding fast in many directions, all of which show promise. Two or three of them will surely be significant forward steps in its diagnosis and treatment. Looking back, it is amazing how far we have come in the last ten years or so. That momentum is picking up, not slowing down. If I am still here to write another edition of this book in, say, five years' time, I am sure it will need a lot of revision, if not a complete re-write.

Glossary

5-alpha-reductase An enzyme that converts testosterone into the more active DHT (see below).

5-alpha-reductase inhibitors Drugs that block the effects of 5-alpha-reductase, thereby shrinking the prostate. One is finasteride.

Androgens Male sex hormone. Formed by the testes and the adrenal glands. They stimulate the growth of prostate cells, normal or cancerous.

Androstene and androstenedione Two male sex hormones produced by the adrenal glands.

Anti-androgens Drugs that neutralize the effects of androgens on the prostate.

BPH Benign Prostatic Hypertrophy or Hyperplasia A benign (non-cancerous) enlargement of the prostate gland.

Brachytherapy Use of radioactive implants (or 'seeds') to treat prostate cancer.

DHT Dihydrotestosterone The most active male sex hormone, closely related to testosterone.

DRE Digital rectal examination Use of the finger to feel the prostate gland from the rectum.

Gleason score A method of assessing the potential malignancy of a cancer under the microscope.

LHRH agonists Drugs that act as anti-androgens, but only after a short androgenic phase.

LHRH antagonists A class of drugs that are anti-androgens without an initial androgenic phase.

Metastases Spread of areas of cancer to distant parts of the body.

Oestrogens Female sex hormone. Can be used as an anti-androgen.

Oncogenes Genes that predispose their possessor to cancer.

Prostatectomy Surgical removal of the prostate.

PSA Prostate specific antigen A substance produced only by prostate gland cells. Used as a 'marker' in the blood for prostate cancer activity.

Radiotherapy Use of radiation to destroy prostate cancers. Given either as an external beam or as implanted seeds.

Testosterone A male sex hormone formed in the testes.

TRUS Trans-urethral ultrasound Use of an ultrasound scan to determine the size of the prostate gland and possible tumours in it.

TURP Trans-urethral resection of the prostate An operation to remove most of the prostate in BPH. Not applicable to prostate cancer.

Urethra The tube that carries urine from the bladder and the ejaculate from the prostate gland out through the penis.

References

Adami, S., *Journal of Urology*, 1985, vol. 134.

Altwein, J. E. *et al.*, *Incidental Cancer of the Prostate*. Springer-Verlag, Berlin, 1991.

Andriole, G. L., *Journal of Urological Abstracts*, 1994, vol. 151.

Armenian, N. K. *et al.*, *Lancet*, 1974, vol. 2.

Bruchovsky, N. *et al.*, *Vitamins and Hormones*, 1975, vol. 33.

Cannon, L., and Bishop, D. T., Cancer Survey, 1982, vol. 1.

Carter, H. B. *et al.*, *Journal of Urology*, 1990, vol. 143.

Chodak, G. W. *et al.*, *New England Journal of Medicine*, 1994a, vol. 330.

Chodak, G. W. *et al.*, *New England Journal of Medicine*, 1994b, vol. 334(4).

Crawford, E. D., *Urology*, 1994, vol. 44.

de Vere White, R. W. *et al.*, *Journal of Urology*, 1993, vol. 149.

DiSilverio, F., *Urology*, 1990, vol. 80.

Drachenberg, D. E., and Brawer, M. K., *Comprehensive Textbook of Genitourinary Oncology*, second edn. Lippincott, Williams & Wilkins, 2000.

Feldman, D. *et al.*, *Experimental Medical Biology*, 1996, vol. 375.

Giovannucci, E. *et al.*, *the US Health Professionals Study, Journal of the National Cancer Institute*, 1993a, vol. 85.

Giovannucci, E. *et al.*, *Journal of the American Medical Association*, 1993b, vol. 269.

Gleave, M. E. *et al.*, *Urology*, 1996, vol. 46.

Goldenberg, S. L., *Journal of Urology*, 1994, vol. 151.

Gonder, M. H., *Investigational Urology*, 1964, vol. 1.

Greenwald, P. *et al.*, *Journal of the National Cancer Institute*, 1974, vol. 5.

Gu, F. L. *et al.*, *Urology*, 1994, vol. 44.

Hanks, G., *Acta Oncologica*, 1991, vol. 30(2).

Heinonen, O. P. *et al.*, *Journal of the National Cancer Institute*, 1998, vol. 90.

Hill, P. B., and Wynder, E.L., *Cancer Letters*, 1979, vol.7.

Kabalin, J. *et al.*, *Journal of Urology*, 1989, vol. 142.

Kirby, R. S., *Reviews of Endocrine-related Cancer*, 1994, vol. 42.

Kirby, R. S., *Prostate*, 1999, vol. 40.

Kirby, R. S., Christmas, T., and Brawer, M., *Prostate Cancer*, second edn. Mosby, 2001.

Labrie, F., *Journal of Steroid Biochemistry*, 1985, vol. 23.

Lancet, Editorial, 1994, vol. 344.

Lee, C. T., and Oesterling, J. E., *Urological Clinics of North America*, 1997, vol. 24(2).

Levran, Z. *et al.*, *British Journal of Urology*, 1995, vol. 75.

Miller, J. I. *et al.*, *Journal of Urology*, 1992, vol. 147.

Myers, C., *Journal of Clinical Oncology*, 1992, vol. 10.

Partin, A. *et al.*, *Journal of Urology*, 1990, vol. 143.

Pasteau, O. and Degrais, P., *Archives of Roentgen Ray*, 1914, vol. 18.

PCTCG, *Lancet*, 1995, vol. 346.

Pilepich, M. V., *American Journal of Clinical Oncology*, 1990, vol. 13.

Pilepich, M. V., *Urology*, 1995, vol. 45.

Porter, A. T., *Seminars in Oncology*, 1993, vol. 20(2).

Ragde, H. *et al.*, *Cancer*, 1998, vol. 83(5).

Rosenberg, L., and Palmer, J. R., *American Journal of Epidemiology*, 1990, vol. 132.

Roth, B. J., *Cancer*, 1993, vol. 72(8).

Sander, S., and Beisland, H. O., *Journal of Urology*, 1984, vol. 132.

Scardino, P. T., *Urological Clinics of North America*, 1989, vol. 16.

Schmid, H. P. *et al.*, *Cancer*, 1993, vol. 71(6).

Schwartz, G. G., and Hulka, B.S., *Anticancer Research*, 1990, vol. 10.

Servadio, C., and Leib, Z., *Urology*, 1991, vol. 38.

Sheldon, C. A., Williams, R. D., and Fraley, E. E., *Journal of Urology*, 1980, vol. 124.

Sidney, S., *Journal of Urology*, 1987, vol. 138.

Smith, J. A., *Journal of Urology*, 1991, vol. 145.

Soloway, M. S. *et al.*, *Journal of Urology*, 1995, vol. 154.

Stamey, T. A., *Monographs in Urology*, 1982, vol. 3.

Stamey, T. A. *et al.*, *Journal of Urology*, 1998, vol. 160(6).

Stanford, J. L. *et al.*, *Journal of the National Cancer Institute*, 1999, vol. 8.

Stein, A. *et al.*, *Journal of Urology*, 1992, vol. 147.

Steinberg, G. S., Carter, B. S., Beaty, T. H. *et al.*, *Prostate*, 1990, vol. 17.

Tretli, S. *et al.*, *Journal of the National Cancer Institute*, 1996, vol. 88.

REFERENCES

Wallner, K. E., *International Journal of Radiation Oncology, Biology and Physiology*, 1996, vol. 14.

Witjes, W. P. J. *et al.*, 'European Organization for Research and Treatment of Cancer (EORTC) Trial', *Urology*, 1997, vol. 49.

Woolf, C. M., *Cancer*, 1960, vol. 13.

Index